Kale

The Complete Guide to the World's Most Powerful Superfood

STEPHANIE PEDERSEN, MS, CHHC

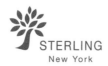

STERLING
New York

STERLING
New York

An Imprint of Sterling Publishing
387 Park Avenue South
New York, NY 10016

ISBN 978-1-4549-0625-4

Distributed in Canada by Sterling Publishing
c/o Canadian Manda Group, 165 Dufferin Street
Toronto, Ontario, Canada M6K 3H6
Distributed in the United Kingdom by GMC Distribution Services
Castle Place, 166 High Street, Lewes, East Sussex, England BN7 1XU
Distributed in Australia by Capricorn Link (Australia) Pty. Ltd.
P.O. Box 704, Windsor, NSW 2756, Australia

For information about custom editions, special sales, and premium and corporate purchases,
please contact Sterling Special Sales at 800-805-5489 or specialsales@sterlingpublishing.com.

Manufactured in the United States of America

2 4 6 8 10 9 7 5 3 1

www.sterlingpublishing.com

PRODUCED BY
AUTHORSCAPE INC.

CONTENTS

Introduction 4

Chapter 1: Getting Friendly With Kale 8

Chapter 2: Kale: The Nutrient Powerhouse 14

Chapter 3: Drink Your Kale! 32

Chapter 4: Breakfast: Start Your Day With Kale 50

Chapter 5: Kale for Lunch 80

Chapter 6: Small Bites: Kale Appetizers and Snacks 104

Chapter 7: Kale for Dinner 120

Chapter 8: Desserts & Other Sweets 142

Chapter 9: Frequently Asked Questions 156

Chapter 10: Kale-Growing Guide 168

Resources 174

Index 184

About the Author 190

Acknowledgments 191

I came late to kale. My Danish cousins ate it in Aunt Jensen's grønkålssuppe. My friends from Scotland and Wales and Ireland and Sweden and Germany and Poland and Russia grew up eating it. Thousands of generations of European peasants, soldiers, artisans, royalty, merchants, men, women, and children were nourished by it.

But me? I was an adult before I even laid eyes on the leafy stuff. That may be because I spent my early years in Australia and California, surrounded by non-leafy vegetables. Or, it could be that, like many children of the 1970s and '80s, the only vegetables I ate came from a can and were usually green beans, peas, peas 'n carrots, tomato sauce, or beetroots, with the occasional fresh cob of corn or head of iceberg lettuce.

My first hands-on experience with kale came when I was in my 20s and working in New York City as a kitchen assistant at the Natural Gourmet Institute, the renowned whole foods cooking school where revolutionary natural foods chefs such as Peter Brearley, Myra Kornfield, Elliot Praag, and Dianne Carlson taught.

Kitchen assistants are the people who help cooking instructors get ready for a class by prepping the ingredients and doing the backstage work during a cooking class. That particular day, a note was waiting for me and two others: "Wash and dry all bunches of kale." Despite a childhood spent tending my parents' berry patch and fruit trees, I couldn't identify which of the gorgeous leafy bundles in front of me was kale.

I turned to another assistant, who shrugged. The third assistant, also unsure, shook his head. Finally, the chef wandered in, saw our confusion, and gave us a quick lesson in kale. The dark, nubbly leaves were Lacinto kale from northern Italy. The tightly ruffled leaves were everyday curly kale. The kale with the magenta rib, was red kale.

Over the course of the next four hours, the three of us eagerly learned how to clean kale, prep it, cook it, and use it. We learned it was one of the most nutrient-dense veggies around and that it was just as good in soups as it was sautéed in coconut or olive oil.

We also learned the subtle differences of the different types. That it tasted sweeter after a frost. That it grew in the Northern Hemisphere.

That it was an ancient member of the cabbage family, more ancient than cabbage itself and the vegetable most other brassica family offspring (such as broccoli and kohlrabi) had descended from. That hippos in the Washington, D.C. zoo ate more than 10 pounds of kale each per day. That the Irish made something called colcannon out of it.

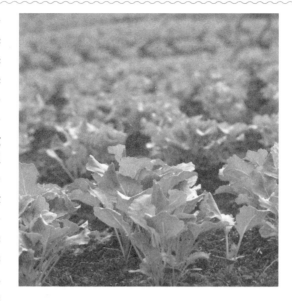

Wanting to get every drop of wisdom we could on this new-to-us veggie, we assigned one of us to take frantic notes while the other two of us worked the kitchen.

After that class, I headed for the farmer's market to stock up, then to the library to check out every cookbook I could find that contained kale recipes. I tried a different kale recipe nearly every day, all the while thanking my luck for having a husband who likes kale! After two months, I got bored. Attempting to shake things up, I began writing some of my own kale recipes.

I adored the way this mighty brassica tasted—bitter and smoky, pungent and slightly sour. Deeply earthy and nourishing. I loved its meaty texture. I was in awe of the omega-3 fatty acids, fiber, phytonutrients, vitamins, minerals, and all of the other good things this leafy green contains. The vegetable felt substantial and fortifying.

What all this experimentation showed me is that kale is gloriously versatile. I began using kale as the basis of vegan, vegetarian, and non-vegetarian main dishes. I started to garnish with kale. I use it today as a salad, as a side veggie, as a snack, and in drinks and soups and sauces. I have even been known to use it in a floral arrangement, as a centerpiece, and as packing material (the curly leaf is best for this!).

Along the way, I learned a few wonderful things firsthand:

- Kale can make your skin look phenomenal, due to its high content of skin-beautifying omega-3 fatty acids, antioxidants, and vitamins A, C, and E. I was no longer experiencing monthly breakouts, my crow's feet softened, and some of the sunspots on my face faded or disappeared.
- Kale provides a sustained energy and increased physical stamina, due to the omega-3 fatty acids.

- Kale helps joints feel better and promotes faster healing between sessions of heavy exercise, thanks to vitamin K, omega-3 fatty acids, and an outstanding number of anti-inflammatory flavonoids. For me, this meant I could go running four days a week without pain.
- Kale's generous fiber content fills the tummy, which left me feeling so satisfied I wasn't interested in after-meal snacking.
- The high beta-carotene content has been linked with improved eyesight. My own fuzzy low-light sight improved after two weeks of eating kale on a daily basis.
- Improved immune system function. Before adding kale to my diet, I caught one cold every four to six weeks. After eating a serving of kale each day, I caught two colds during an entire year. The veggie's antioxidant content is the reason.
- While I don't have personal experience with the following conditions, my kale research uncovered mountains of studies on kale's numerous nutrients and how they help prevent and heal heart conditions, high cholesterol, cancer, and diseases of the gall bladder and liver.

And, perhaps most important to my personal life, kale also helps your body powerfully and quickly get rid of toxins and old wastes.

Pregnant during the 9/11 World Trade Center attacks, I was exposed to a massive amount of toxins. I passed these on to my son, who was born with off-the-charts levels of heavy metal poisoning.

It took me a few years to learn that heavy metal poisoning was behind my child's perplexing symptoms (a complex mix of skin, digestive, sensory, sleep, and mood disorders). Once I got to the bottom of his health crisis, I began working hard to rebuild his immune system and naturally and gently detox his small body. Kale puree was one of our mainstays. I hid it in smoothies and marinara sauce. I made green eggs and mashed potatoes. I minced kale leaves into soup and meatballs and pots of brown rice, millet, and quinoa.

I increased my own kale intake to help rid myself of the metals I'd acquired while pregnant. Today, we're both clean and healthy, in large part due to this ancient food's super healing abilities.

Kale is indeed a "superfood," and a popular one at that. While it hasn't yet surpassed potatoes as America's favorite vegetable, you can check out any raw food blog, vegan restaurant, vegetarian magazine, or alternative health Web site and find "unofficial proof" that kale is the darling of the health set.

I have my own unofficial proof that kale is the health world's most popular vegetable: At one point in my career I worked as a writer for the Institute of Integrative Nutrition in New York City. One of my duties was to compose alumni bios for the school's Web site. I would send each IIN graduate a questionnaire, read through their answers, edit them, and post the answers online for other people to see. When asked "What is your favorite health food?", 195 out of about 200 people said "kale."

Just to make my proof a little more official: I began quizzing my nutritionist and natural chef friends. My alternative healer friends. My acupuncturist, massage therapist, chiropractor, Reiki healer, and several personal trainers. Yoginis. Raw foodists. Feng shui masters. Vitamin supplement peddlers.

People standing behind me in the Whole Foods' checkout line.

Every single one of them had the same favorite vegetable: Kale.

I suppose I could have found more people to ask, but the above was enough for me. In my opinion, kale is the country's favorite superfood. For so many reasons.

Keep reading to learn what these reasons are!

Love and kale chips to you all,
Stephanie Pedersen, MS, CHHC AADP
Holistic Nutritionist

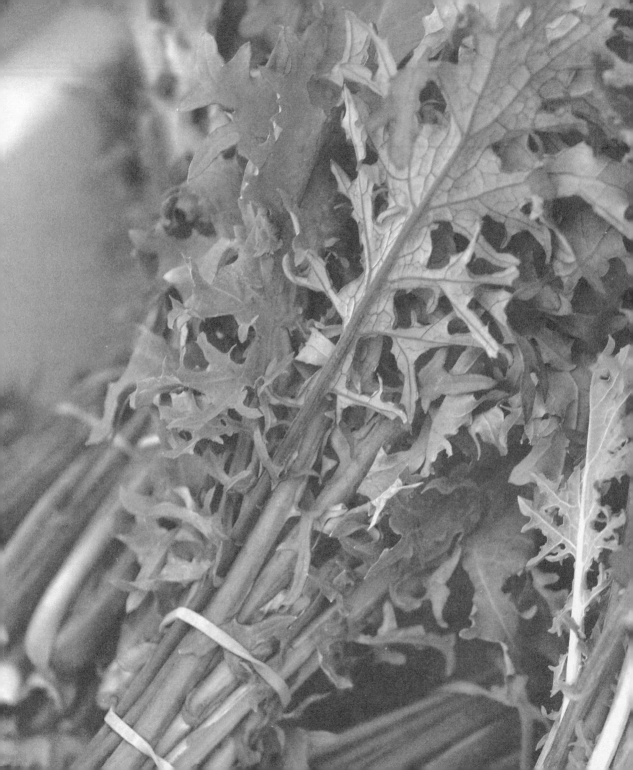

CHAPTER 1

GETTING FRIENDLY WITH KALE

Hello kale lovers! I am so excited to share my favorite veggie with like-minded foodies. And welcome, also, to you healthy folks who have heard that kale is a great way to uplevel your health. And lastly, friendly greetings to those of you out there who cannot stand kale, but are here because you love someone who loves kale, or your doctor or nutritionist told you that you need to be eating more green veggies, or you want to make sure your family gets the greens they need to be their best.

Kale comes in several colors, sizes, and leaf styles, including the popular curly (also known as ruffled or frilled); the shiny, smooth leaves (such as Lacinto kale); and the red-hued, lobed leaves (such as red Russian kale). By all means experiment with the different types. You may be like me and love all varieties equally. Or, you may find you prize one type above the rest. All have near-identical nutritional profiles and that green, earthy taste you expect from kale. All can be used interchangeably in kale recipes. And all should be chosen and stored following the same guidelines.

For those of you who prefer tender, mild-tasting kale, opt for bunches with smaller-sized leaves, which are younger and less fibrous than their larger, more mature siblings. Note that although kale is now available throughout the year, the sweetest, mildest greens are available during the plant's peak, which is from winter through the beginning of spring.

KALE'S ILLUSTRIOUS HISTORY

Wild kale was first found growing in cool, sandy soil in the Eastern Mediterranean (though some researchers say Asia Minor was kale's first home). Early kale was a scraggly, leggy plant. As humans became aware of its deliciousness and its ability to create and maintain health, they began seeking the plant out, gathering its seeds and planting their own stash of kale. They also began trading the seeds with people of other regions and carrying the plant through other lands in the rations of soldiers and explorers, spreading the plant up into Europe and the British Isles, over to Russia, and even across the sea to North America.

Regardless of the size of leaves or varieties you choose, however, one of the best, most foolproof ways to be sure your loved ones (you included!) eat their weekly servings of kale is to start with the best quality kale you can. The first step in doing that is to "eat fresh."

Curly leaves or smooth leaves, green leaves or red leaves, whether you're in the supermarket or farmer's market, look for kale with spry, bouncy leaves. Yes, I did just say "spry." I know it sounds strange, but you'll know what I mean when you see a bunch of kale. Avoid kale with any slimy spots, a yellow tinge (or bright yellowing of the leaves), or greens with dried-out stem ends. Further, you do not want wilted or dehydrated or shriveled-looking kale. Here's why:

Kale and other veggies wilt when they lose moisture. For those science aficionados out there, this happens because as moisture evaporates from the veggie, its cell walls lose rigidity. The vegetables become soft and flexible. As unappetizing as a wilted veggie is, there is an even bigger issue at hand: As moisture leaves the plant, it takes nutrients with it. Moisture loss not only reduces vitamin C and A levels, it also contributes to yellowing and bitterness. This means that the more flabby and dehydrated a kale leaf is, the less nutrients and taste it contains. And that's a problem.

KALE THEN AND NOW

The kale we grow today is almost identical to the kale that tribes foraged thousands of years ago. The prime difference is that now the leaves are bigger. The change in leaf size happened over many seasons as people who cultivated kale saved leaves from the plant that had the largest leaves. Meet the seed for next year's crop! Repeat this process over hundreds of years, maybe longer, and you will end up with large-leafed kale.

If you grow your own kale (see Chapter 10 if you'd like to try this yourself), allow kale to stay in the garden until you plan to use it. Otherwise, place kale in the fridge as soon as you get it home. Several studies have shown that kale loses up to 89 percent of its vitamin C when left at 70°F (the typical temperature in a transport truck or even a vase of water on the kitchen counter, something many chefs unfortunately suggest) for two days after picking, compared to 5 percent for kale stored at just above freezing for that same period.

As for washing beforehand, don't: Washing kale before storage encourages spoilage *and* it hastens nutrient loss. So wrap it or bag it and place it in the fridge. Although you can store kale for up to five days if it was superfresh when purchased, I'd personally use it sooner. Not only will it lose important nutrients the longer it hangs out in your fridge, the more bitter its flavor will become. This is not a good thing for kids, or other veggiephobes. If you notice the leaves yellowing, toss it: Not only will the flavor be too strong, the nutrients will be almost nil.

> Brassica oleracea is the Latin name for kale. Brassica, the genus name, meaning *cabbage family*, and olacerea, the species name, meaning *without a head*. Soon, variations cropped up; some seeds sprouted into kale with large smooth leaves, or that bunched together or flowered at the top, or had engorged roots or swollen nodes at its base or stalk. Soon, people were saving seeds of these variants, which came to be known, respectively, as collards, cabbage, broccoli, rutabaga, turnip, kohlrabi, and Brussels' sprouts—all grandchildren of wild kale.

Another nutrient no-no: Pre-prepping your kale, then stashing it in the fridge until you have time to cook with it. Cooking magazines, mommy blogs, and television chefs champion the practice of prepping veggies in the fridge to encourage healthy nibbling and easier weeknight cooking. In theory, the idea is awesome: Open the fridge, grab whatever prepped bit of produce you need, and voila:

A healthy, convenient, economical snack. If, after you read what I have to say on the subject, you still want to pre-prep your kale, go ahead. Eating pre-prepped kale is so much better than eating no kale at all! But do hear me out: Pre-cut fruits and veggies lose between 10 to 25 percent of their vitamin C and carotenoids. That's because oxygen destroys antioxidants. When kale (or any produce) is cut, the cut area is instantly exposed to oxygen, starting the breakdown of nutrients. Precooking kale (or other veggies and fruit) to use at a later time also saps nutrients.

So, how to store your kale so you get the most nutrient dense veggie possible? Again, don't wash it, for starters! Remove any wilted or yellowed or spotty bits, then place your kale in a storage bag, first removing as much air from the bag as possible before tightly fastening shut. Store the bag in the vegetable crisper section of the refrigerator for no more than five days.

> ### KALE BY ANY OTHER NAME...
>
> Kale is often called "borecole" in some English-speaking countries. "Kale" is a Scottish word derived from *coles* or *caulis*, terms used by the Greeks and Romans in referring to the whole cabbage-like group of plants. The German word *kohl* has the same origin.

If you are nearing day four and you still haven't used your kale, you are in the perfect place! Simply check out one of the recipes in this book and head to the kitchen!

No time to cook? Go ahead and wash the kale, then de-rib it by folding the leaf together and pulling out the center rib. No need for a knife! This can be done entirely by hand. Next, place a large pot of water on the stove. When the water is boiling, blanch the de-ribbed kale by submerging it in the boiling water for two to three minutes. Immediately place the kale in a bowl or colander and run very cold water over it until the kale is cool to the touch. Tuck it into an airtight container and place in the fridge to use within two or three days or freeze it immediately for up to a month. You can defrost the kale and add it to soups, pasta, casseroles, and other dishes.

DID YOU KNOW…?

You may hear kale being labeled as a member of the cruciferous family. What is this family and how is it different than the brassica family everyone lumps kale into? Well, actually they're the same family. At one point, botanists referred to the group as *Cruciferous*, a Latin word meaning "cross-bearing." This described the four petals of mustard flowers—one of kale's cousins—which are reminiscent of a cross.

THE TALE OF TWO KALES

When you shop for kale, you will notice that the veggie sports various types of leaf shapes. That's because there are two kinds of kale, Brassica napus and Brassica oleraceae. Brassica napus is the curly or ruffled-leaf kale, and includes the Pabularia group known as Siberian kale or red Russian kale.

Brassica oleraceae is the smoother-leaved family, including the Acephala group, which features collards and dinosaur kale. Dinosaur kale is a much more recent variety. It was discovered in Italy in the late 19th century.

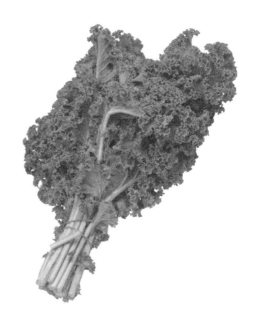

KALE'S ENORMOUS PLANT FAMILY

Kale is a member of the brassica family, an insanely diverse family with thousands of relatives. The *Cambridge World History of Food* cites 400 types of one relative, the cabbage, alone. It is estimated that there are more than 78,000 samples of the major brassicas and their wild relatives (inelegantly called "weeds") in more than 130 countries throughout the world. Here is just a sampling of kale's many cousins:

- Horseradish
- Land cress
- Ethiopian mustard
- Collard greens
- Chinese broccoli (Gai-Lan)
- Cabbage
- Brussels sprout
- Kohlrabi
- Broccoli
- Broccoflower
- Broccoli romanesco
- Cauliflower brassica
- Wild broccoli
- Bok choy
- Komatsuna
- Mizuna
- Rapini (Broccoli rabe)
- Flowering cabbage brassica
- Chinese cabbage (Napa cabbage)

- Turnip root / turnip greens
- Rutabaga
- Siberian kale
- Canola / rapeseed
- Wrapped heart mustard cabbage
- Mustard greens
- Mustard seed, brown
- Mustard seeds, white
- Mustard seeds, black
- Tatsoi
- Arugula / rocket / roquette
- Field pepperweed
- Maca
- Garden cress
- Watercress
- Radish
- Daikon
- Wasabi

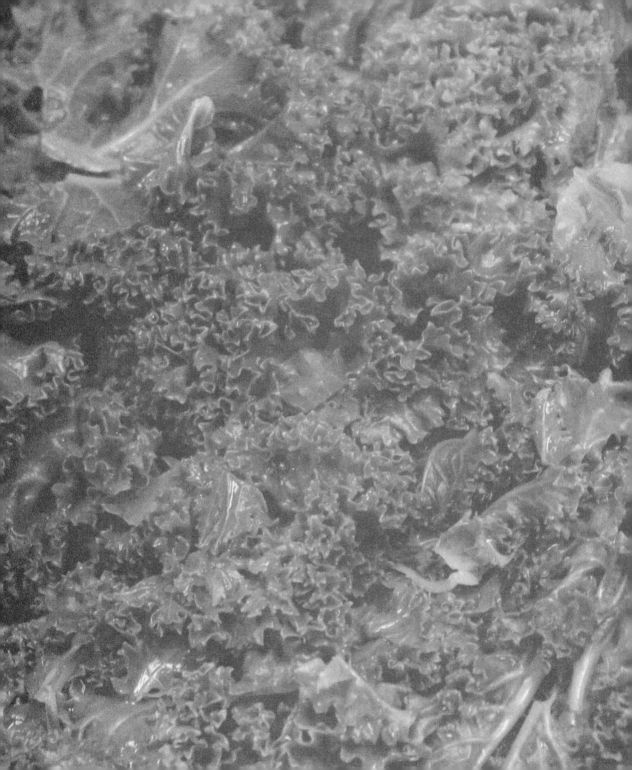

CHAPTER 2

KALE: THE NUTRIENT POWERHOUSE

Kale tastes great. It's versatile, straight-forward to cook, and easy to find. But it's kale's nutrient profile that makes it the darling of the healthy-living set. With dozens of vitamins and as many minerals, plus fiber, antioxidants, fatty acids, amino acids, and protein, kale is the veggie world's most-valuable-player.

For maximum health benefits, plan to eat kale at least three times a week (more often is even better!), enjoying anywhere from one cup to two cups at a time. Because different nutrients become available for the body to use in different concentrations when kale is eaten raw, lightly cooked or long-simmered, try to enjoy your greens in a variety of ways so that your body gets a hefty dose of everything.

For a deeper look at the nutrients kale offers—and what it can do for your health—keep reading. I think you'll be very impressed.

VITAMIN A

Kale is loaded with the plant-source form of vitamin A, called beta carotene (the form of vitamin A from animal-source food is called a retinoid). One cup of cooked kale contains an outrageous 17707.30 IU of vitamin A, which equals 354.1 percent of an adult's daily recommended allowance of the nutrient. This means enjoying kale a few times a week is a super way to ensure your body gets the vitamin A it needs.

VITAMIN A: WHAT HAPPENS WHEN THERE IS NOT ENOUGH

While most of us get plenty of vitamin A, deficiencies in this important vitamin are not uncommon. This is especially true for chronic dieters, those living on processed food, and individuals suffering from food scarcity. Here's what a lack of vitamin A can cause:

- Night blindness. This is one of the first signs of vitamin A deficiency
- Dry eyes, also known as Xerophthalmia
- Complete blindness
- Maternal mortality in pregnant women
- Miscarriage
- Inability to breast feed
- Increased risk of catching infection diseases
- Retarded or decreased childhood growth
- Slow bone development in children

Why this is important: Vitamin A has been shown to protect the body against cancer and it is a potent anti-inflammatory ingredient. It softens premature aging (including wrinkles, sun spots, and slack skin), wards off asthma, helps knock out pneumonia, and fights candida, heart disease, and inflammatory conditions such as arthritis and heart disease. It strengthens the immune system by helping the body fend off virus, bacterial attacks, and other illnesses. It improves photosensitivity and fertility, and fights macular degeneration. It even helps improve the bio-availability of iron and zinc in the body and prevent low birth-weight babies. How's that for a wide range of benefits?

VITAMIN B1

Vitamin B1, also known as thiamin, was the first of the B vitamins to be discovered. (The B vitamins—known collectively as B-complex vitamins—are a group of eight related water soluble nutrients.) Its discovery was a bit of an accident. Dutch doctor and medical researcher Christiaan Eijkman was studying beriberi patients in Jakarta when he realized that people who ate brown rice (which still has its bran coating intact) didn't get the disease. Upon closer study and after conducting several research trials, Eijkman was able to identify a nutrient contained in brown rice that he later named Vitamin B. This substance seemed to protect people from beriberi.

The vitamin works wonders in maintaining nervous system and muscle health, as well as helping the body convert sugar to usable energy.

Brown rice, seeds, and legumes (such as lentils and beans) are terrific sources of vitamin B1. With each serving containing .07 mg of vitamin B1, 4.9 percent of an adult's daily recommended allowance, kale does not contain as much vitamin B1 as these sources, but it is a good, easy way to add thiamin to your daily diet.

STUTTERING BE GONE!

Did you know there are approximately 68 million people worldwide who stutter, most of them males? (Males are 4 times as likely to stutter as females.) Fortunately, there is help. One is vitamin B1, a vitamin also known as thiamine that is found in kale. Numerous studies have found the B-vitamin helpful in lessening or even eradicating adult stuttering. One of the most recent, completed by the National Center for Stuttering in 2011, followed 38 male stutterers, ages 21 to 37, for two weeks. One group received 300 mg of vitamin B1 daily, while the other group received a placebo. The placebo group showed no improvement through the course of the trial, while in the vitamin B1 group, something curious happened: Everybody in the vitamin group showed some improvement, and one-third of them were completely cured. Even after a seven-month follow-up, the stutter-free men still had not returned to stuttering.

VITAMIN B2: DID YOU KNOW...?

- Riboflavin has been shown to lessen the severity of and decrease the number of migraine headaches a person has.
- Drinking caffeinated beverages can deplete vitamin B2 (as well as other important nutrients such as magnesium and vitamins A, B1, B3, and B5).
- Ariboflavinosis is the official term for vitamin B2 deficiency.
- A deficiency of vitamin B2 can cause cracked skin in the corners of the mouth, chapped lips, and soreness and inflammation of the mouth and tongue.
- Vitamin B2 deficiency can lead to cataracts.
- Children who do not get enough vitamin B2 may experience retarded growth.
- Sugar depletes the body's store of vitamin B2, as well as all other B-complex vitamins.
- People who are often fatigued and lethargic are frequently also low in vitamin B2.
- Riboflavin helps the body metabolize iron, making the vitamin an important nutrient for those suffering from iron-deficiency anemia.
- Hypersensitivity to light can be a sign of a vitamin B2 deficiency.

VITAMIN B2

Known alternately as riboflavin and vitamin B2, this special nutrient plays several roles, including helping the body to maintain its supply of other B-complex vitamins, protecting the cells from oxygen damage and supporting cellular energy production. It also helps to prevent and treat anemia, carpal tunnel syndrome, cataracts, dry eyes, eye conditions including sensitivity to light and blurry vision, recurring headaches (including migraines), rosacea, and skin rashes.

Kale is a good source of this important vitamin. I've got to be completely honest: kale does not contain the extreme riboflavin levels that cremini mushrooms, spinach, and venison do, but one cup of our favorite brassica provides .09 mg, or 5.3 percent of an adult's daily recommended allowance for vitamin B2. Kale is an easy, yummy way to get more of this essential B-complex vitamin into your diet.

VITAMIN B3

You may know vitamin B3 by its other name: Niacin. Like its B-complex cousins, niacin helps the body with energy production at a cellular level. It is also necessary to sustain healthy levels of cholesterol, stabilize blood sugar, help the body process fats, and help the cells create new DNA.

VITAMIN B3: DID YOU KNOW…?

- Niacin was first discovered by chemist Hugo Weidel in 1873 in his studies of nicotine.
- Vitamin B3's original name, nicotinic acid, was changed to niacin (*nicotinic acid + vitamin*) to disassociate it from nicotine.
- Symptoms of vitamin B3 deficiency include: aggression, dermatitis, diarrhea, insomnia, intolerance of cold, mental confusion, and physical weakness. Late-stage conditions associated with vitamin B3 deficiency include pellagra.
- In the 1930s, vitamin B3 was also called Pellagra-Preventing Factor, as it was essential in preventing and curing pellagra.
- Foods rich in vitamin B3 include: brewer's yeast, broccoli, carrots, cheese, dandelion greens, dates, eggs, fish, kale, milk, peanuts, potatoes, tomatoes, tuna, veal, beef liver, and chicken breast.
- Niacin was named vitamin B3 because it was the third of the B vitamins to be discovered.
- Another name for vitamin B3 is vitamin PP.
- Vegemite, the Australian spread made of barley-based brewer's yeast extract, is one of the highest sources of niacin. A 5-gram serving contains 25 percent of an adult's daily recommended intake of the vitamin.

That's a lot of important jobs for one nutrient! Don't get enough vitamin B3 and you may feel tired and lethargic—you may even experience muscle weakness, digestive upset, or skin rashes.

Kale contains moderate amounts of most B-complex vitamins, including vitamin B3. One cup of cooked kale contains .65 mg of niacin, which is 3.2 percent of an adult's daily recommended allowance. Every little bit counts!

VITAMIN B6

When vitamin B6 was first discovered in 1934, it was called Antidermatitis Factor for its role in preventing and healing skin conditions, such as general inflammation, dermatitis, psoriasis, and eczema. It also helps the body heal cardiovascular disease, carpal tunnel syndrome, depression, diabetic neuropathy—it has even been shown to improve autism and epilepsy conditions, as well as alleviate the effects of alcoholism, adrenal gland dysfunction, asthma, HIV/AIDS, kidney stones, PMS, and vaginitis. Vitamin B6 has also been used to reduce pregnancy-related nausea, prevent brain shrinkage in Alzheimer's patients, lower the risk of lung cancer, and even to help break

WHAT ARE OXALATES AND WHY ARE THEY IN KALE?

As much good stuff as kale has, it also contains something that a few people may want to watch out for: Oxalates. These naturally-occurring molecules are organic acids, and they are made by most all living things, plant and animal. Humans regularly convert substances, such as vitamin C, to oxalates. For most people, oxalates are a neutral substance that doesn't affect health. But for others, oxalates can become a problem if there are too many of them in the body. Excess oxalates can crystallize in the gallbladder or kidneys, leading to gallstones or kidney stones. To stay on the safe side, restrict your consumption of high-oxalate foods, such as spinach, and aim for no more than one to two servings of cooked or raw kale per week.

up kidney stones. With all that, it's no wonder that vitamin B6 is the most thoroughly studied of the B-complex vitamins.

Luckily for you, every time you eat kale, you are getting a good amount of this wonder nutrient. One cup of cooked kale gives you .18 mg of B6, which equals 9 percent of an adult's daily recommended allowance. As if you needed another reason to eat kale!

SWEETER DREAMS WITH B6

A 2002 study at the City College of New York suggests that 250 mg of vitamin B6 a day increases one's dream vividness and the ability to recall dreams. The explanation for this phenomena is that vitamin B6 increases sleeptime arousal during periods of rapid eye movement (REM) sleep.

VITAMIN B9

If you are a woman of childbearing age, have been a woman of childbearing age, or know a woman of childbearing age, you may know vitamin B9 by its other names: Folate, or folic acid. This is the nutrient obstetricians and midwifes urge their patients to take starting the moment they are considering having a baby.

Here's why: Folate gets a lot of attention for helping to prevent birth defects, specifically those involving the neural tube (the body part that later forms the brain and spinal column) and the cleft palate. It has also been found to reduce the risk of nervous system disorders in infants, help ward off Alzheimer's disease and dementia, prevent osteoporosis, and lower the risk of cancers of the esophagus and lung, uterus, cervix, and intestine. Folate also keeps skin dermatitis-free.

THE HIGH COST OF FOLIC ACID DEFICIENCY

Every year, about 3,000 babies in the United States are born with spina bifida or anenceph-aly. These neural tube defects are caused by the incomplete closing of the fetus's spine and skull during pregnancy. The total lifetime cost of care for a child born with spina bifida is estimated to be $560,000. The annual medical care and surgical costs for people with spina bifida exceed $200 million. These expenditures are nothing compared to the emotional heartache connected with the condition. What's especially sad is 50 to 70 percent of these neural tube defects could be prevented if women took just 400 mcg of folic acid daily, before and during pregnancy.

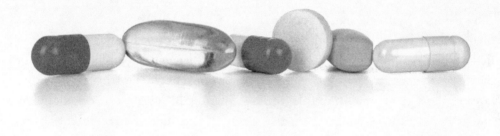

Vitamin B9 is another B-complex vitamin that is available in moderate amounts in kale. One cup of the cooked greens contains 16.90 mcg, or 3.6 percent of an adult's daily allowance for the nutrient.

VITAMIN C

Vitamin C was the first-discovered—and remains one of the best known—of anti-oxidant vitamins, meaning it fights oxidation in the body. You probably already know what oxidation is: Think of a cut apple. What happens when its flesh is exposed to air; It gets brown, right? That's oxidation.

A small bit of oxidation happens naturally in the body during regular cell function. But unsafe levels of oxidation can occur when you are exposed to steady amounts of pollution, chemicals, processed food, excess sugar, alcohol, cigarette smoke, and even stress. The result is cell damage and even death. Oxidation makes our skin look older, our immunity weaker, and our bodies more prone to fatigue and illness.

Vitamin C, also known as ascorbic acid, can help the body ward off oxidation by a complex chemical reaction that kills oxidized cells. It also helps with wound healing, maintains healthy tissue (from skin tissue to gum tissue to the tissue that makes up our blood vessels), and boosts the immune system. Fortunately, kale is packed with this hardworking nutrient. One cup of our favorite veggie packs 53.30 mg of the vitamin, providing 88.8 percent of an adult's recommended daily allowance.

VITAMIN E

Vitamin E, known in nutritionist circles as tocopherol, is a powerful antioxidant. Actually, it's a powerful *family* of antioxidants—vitamin E is a generic term for a cluster of eight structurally-similar, related molecules that work together to protect the body from oxidative stress, strengthen the immune system, and protect the nervous and cardiovascular systems.

A 1-cup serving of kale can give you 1.11 mg of vitamin E. That's 5.6 percent of an adult's recommended daily allowance. True, that's not a huge amount, but it is a respectable quantity, in a delicious, easily digestible form. And because vitamin E is fat soluble—meaning that it is stored in your body's fat tissue until needed—most people don't need as much vitamin E as they would a water-soluble vitamin in which any extra amount is immediately excreted from the system.

VITAMIN K

There are many people in the world who have never heard of vitamin K. Identified in 1929 by Danish scientist Henrik Dam, the nutrient was named vitamin K after its discovery was mentioned in a German medical journal, which referred to it as *Koagulationsvitamin*.

Vitamin K is perhaps best known for its role in helping blood to clot normally. Many people who are deficient in the vitamin notice that they bruise easily, or experience heavy nose bleeding, excessive bleeding from everyday cuts, overly-heavy menstrual

VITAMIN K'S BLOOD CLOTTING CONSIDERATION

Vitamin K is essential for helping blood clot quickly and easily in the presence of a wound. But for the thousands of individuals who suffer from cardiovascular conditions and are currently on blood-thinning medication, the natural clotting attributes of vitamin K can be a problem. If you are one of these people, discuss your diet with your health provider before starting to take more vitamin K. Usually, individuals on blood thinners can safely eat kale three or four times a week, whereas vitamin K supplements are strictly off-limits. But as always, discuss with your doctor before you make any changes in your diet or supplement schedule.

bleeding, and even rectal bleeding. But the nutrient also assists with strengthening healthy bones, helping to protect against bone loss and fractures.

Kale is one of the richest dietary sources of vitamin K around—just one cup of the greens contains 1,062.10 mcg of the vitamin, or 1,327.6 percent of an adult's recommended daily allowance of vitamin K.

CAROTENOIDS

Carotenoids are chemicals that exist in plant and animal pigments. In other words, they help give living things their color. While science is still studying carotenoids, as of now 600 different carotenoids have been identified including, beta-carotene, alpha-carotene, gamma-carotene, lycopene, lutein, beta-cryptoxanthin, zeaxanthin, and astaxanthin. Carotenoids happen to be powerful anti-oxidants that protect and strengthen human cells—each carotenoid provides slightly different benefits, but overall, they work to increase immune system function and fight off the damages of free radicals in the body.

Long-term low intake of carotenoids—which is not uncommon among people who don't eat several servings of veggies a day—can make you susceptible to infertility, lowered immunity against infectious diseases, and an increased risk of cardiovascular diseases and cancers. It can also diminish the quality of your skin, hair, and nails.

No current recommended dietary intake levels have been established for carotenoids. However, in order to get adequate carotenoid levels, the United Sates National Academy of Sciences recommends that individuals consume five or more servings of fruits and vegetable (such as kale!) every day.

KALE KEEPS EYES YOUNG

Age-related macular degeneration (known as ARMD) is the world's leading cause of blindness for people 65 and older. It occurs when cells (called macular cells) in the center of the eye's retina begin to deteriorate. Fortunately, kale can help prevent ARMD, as well as slow its progress. The specific nutrients in kale responsible for this feat? Two carotenoids called lutein and zeaxanthin.

As antioxidants, lutein and zeaxanthin help in three ways: By defending the retina against cell-damaging free radicals, by maintaining blood vessels in the macula (so oxygen and other nutrients thus ensuring a constant supply of healing oxygen and nutrients), and by filtering out UV light, which has been found to be damaging to eyesight.

Consider recent evidence: Two separate studies show that eating foods rich in lutein can increase macular pigment. In 1995, The Eye Disease Case-Control Study, conducted at the Massachusetts Eye and Ear Infirmary in Boston, found that individuals with the highest blood levels of lutein and zeaxanthin were 70 percent less likely to develop ARMD than those with the lowest levels. The study also found that people who ate lutein- and zeaxanthin-rich greens (such as kale and spinach) five or more times a week (averaging 6 mg of lutein a day) were 43 percent less likely to suffer from ARMD than those who consumed the greens less than once a month. Moreover, the Harvard Nurses' Health Study, in which nurses (71,494 women and 41,564 men ages 50 years and older) were followed for 18 years through the 1980s and into the '90s, found that eating spinach more than five days a week lowered ARMD risk by 47 percent.

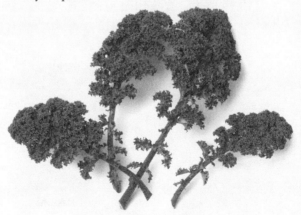

FLAVONOIDS

Flavonoids are plant-based pigments that boast powerful antioxidant benefits. Over 4,000 have been identified and it is believed there may ultimately be between 5,000 to 10,000 flavonoids in existence. Like carotenoids, flavonoids help protect the body's cells from degeneration and damage. In a 2010 research study in the Netherlands, it was found that individuals with the greatest flavonoid intake (30 to 50 mg) had a 20 percent lower risk of stroke than those in the study who had the lowest flavonoid intake. While no dietary recommendations have been set for flavonoids, and few foods have been measured for exact flavonoid amounts, you can easily get 30 to 50 mg of flavonoids in your diet by eating between three to five servings of veggies a day, including kale, which is rich in the nutrient.

FINDING FLAVONOIDS

Originally known only for their roles as plant pigments, no one realized that flavonoids were beneficial until 1938 when a Hungarian scientist named Albert Szent-Gyorgyi—the same researcher who won a Nobel Prize in 1936 for isolating and identifying vitamin C—realized that flavonoids did so much more than create pretty colors.

TOO STINKY FOR BUGS

We humans consider them cancer-fighters, but kale and other brassica-family plants manufacture strong-smelling glucosinolate to repel bugs.

GLUCOSINOLATES

Glucosinolates are phytonutrients. More precisely, they are sulfur-containing compounds that have been shown to have a powerful effect on cancer—both lowering your risk and helping cancer patients beat their illnesses. Glucosinolates also have strong detoxifying effects, helping the body rid itself of potentially dangerous toxins, which can contribute to a number of diseases and brain differences. Lastly, glucosinolates have been shown to have anti-inflammatory abilities, helping the body reduce the cellular inflammation that is tied to a range of illnesses, from heart disease to rheumatoid arthritis.

There is no current recommended daily allowance of glucosinolate, but kale is rich in the nutrient. Eating three or more servings of kale per week is all you need to get the glucosinolate that can help you stay your healthiest.

FIBER

Fiber gives structure to food. In animal protein, it is typically the muscle fiber. In plant food, such as kale, it provides the tell-tale shape of the leaf (or stalk, root, tuber, bulb, flower, pod, or seed). There are a few reasons why fiber is a good thing for humans to eat: First, fiber binds to things—bad things—and helps escort them from the body. Cholesterol is one of these things. Fiber surrounds cholesterol in the blood, basically absorbing it, so it never has to be sent to the liver to be broken down. This helps lower blood cholesterol levels and the amount of cholesterol in the liver

Secondly—and you probably already know about this one—fiber helps promote bowel regularity. Yep, it helps make digestion easier, by surrounding waste in the large intestine and helping carry it out of the body. This prevents constipation and lessens the time intestinal tissue is in contact with waste that may contain carcinogens, thus lessening one's risk of cancer. Another digestive benefit of fiber: Fiber feeds the "friendly" flora in the large intestine, helping keep flora populations strong and healthy so they can break down any poorly digested food that makes its way into the colon.

Fiber also helps keep blood sugar levels low, which is important for diabetics, people with hypoglycemia, and anyone who suffers from food cravings. Fiber does this by slowing the rate at which food (and blood sugar) leaves the stomach after eating. Why this is good: It means a big rush of blood sugar isn't dumped into the blood all at once, which in turn creates

THE TWO TYPES OF FIBER

Fiber is what gives food structure. It comes in two varieties, insoluble and soluble. Insoluble fiber, the type found in kale and brassica-family veggies, does not change, break down or dissolve in the presence of liquids. Soluble fiber (which I call "swellable fiber") is found in things like oats. It softens and swells when it gets wet. You need both for good health.

dangerous spikes in blood sugar, weakness, moodiness, irritability, and cravings.

Those trying to lose weight find diminished cravings helpful in warding off overeating. Plus, fiber creates a feeling of supreme satiety in the stomach, making you feel so full that you don't want to put unneeded food in your system. Voila! Less calories!

Kale contains a good amount of fiber. A 1-cup serving of the cooked green provides 2.60 grams and 10.4 percent of an adult's daily recommended allowance of fiber.

INDIGESTION AID?

It is said that Julius Caesar ate a generous serving of collards as an indigestion preventive after attending royal banquets—a testimony to the green's detoxifying properties! Does this make collards nature's all-natural antacid?

OMEGA-3 FATTY ACIDS

Omega-3 fatty acids are essential in helping a large number of body systems to function efficiently; quickly improve the look and health of skin, hair, and nails; enhance attention and mental acuity; and boost the immune system. They've been found to help the body lose weight and keep it off, guarding against a wide range of health conditions, such as cardiovascular disease, stroke, cancer, inflammatory bowel disease, and immune system diseases such as lupus and rheumatoid arthritis.

Because the body does not produce omega-3 fatty acid molecules on its own, it must get the nutrient through food. Kale can help! One cup of the cooked green contains .13 g, which equals 5.4 percent of an adult's daily recommended allowance for omega-3 fatty acids.

NON-KALE SOURCES OF OMEGA-3 FATTY ACIDS

A serving of these foods provides the following USDA's recommended daily allowance of omega-3 fatty acids:
- Chia seed, 2 tablespoons: 150%
- Flax seed, 2 tablespoons: 132.9%
- Walnuts, ¼ cup: 94.5%
- Salmon, 4 ounces: 61.2%
- Sardines, 4 ounces: 55.8%
- Soybeans, 1 cup: 42.9%
- Halibut, 4 ounces: 25.8%
- Scallops, 4 ounces: 17%
- Shrimp, 4 ounces: 15.4%
- Tuna, 4 ounces: 13.7%

PROTEIN

Protein is one of the most important, and most misunderstood, nutrients in the modern diet. Taken from the Greek word *proteos*, which means "primary" or "taking first place," protein was the first substance to be recognized as a vital part of living tissue. Accounting for 20 percent of our body weight, proteins perform a wide variety of functions throughout the body as vital components of body tissues, enzymes, and immune cells, including production of structural tissue such as muscle, tendons, and skin; production of antibodies, which are used by the immune system to ward off infections; production of enzymes and hormones; and maintenance of the body's proper fluid balance.

Individuals who are pregnant, recovering from physical or emotional illness or trauma, chronic illness sufferers, endurance athletes, physical laborers, and children need more protein than the general population. That said, protein deficiency is rare in the western world—most North Americans and Europeans get more protein than they can use. However, about 300 million children in the developing world are believed to be protein-deficient; 40 percent of them die from increased susceptibility of infections. Deficiency symptoms include muscle weakness, fatigue, hair loss, brain fog, water retention, frequent infections, lowered immune system function, enlarged fatty liver, and muscle wasting.

While most people don't think of leafy greens having much protein, kale has a moderate amount. One cup of cooked greens contains 2.47 grams, or 4.9 percent of an adult's daily recommended allowance of easy-to-digest protein.

COMPLETE VS. INCOMPLETE

When it comes to protein, there are two kinds: complete and incomplete. Complete protein contains all nine essential amino acids. Animal food sources such as meat, fish, poultry, eggs, milk, and cheese that fall in this category are always complete proteins. Other complete proteins are a few plant foods, such as chia, quinoa, buckwheat, amaranth, chlorella, and spirulina. In most cases, however, plant foods are deficient in one or more essential amino acid, making them incomplete proteins. This isn't such a big deal—just eat two of them within the same day (or same meal, such as beans and brown rice, or a millet-kale-nut pilaf), and you'll get the full complement of essential amino acids necessary to create complete protein.

HOW OUR DIETS HAVE CHANGED

Back before electricity, plumbing, and perhaps even before the wheel, humans ate much differently than they do today. One of the most dramatic changes to the human diet has been the ratio between omega-3 and omega-6 essential fatty acids (EFA). Our bodies require both of these essential fatty acids. However modern diets consist of much more omega-6 fatty acids, the fatty acid found in grain-fed poultry and meat, and industrially produced cooking oils, such as safflower and canola oils.

Historically, during the hunter-and-gatherer era, this balance was 1:1 or even 1:2 in favor of omega-3 fatty acids, the fatty acids that protect the nervous and cardiovascular systems, and which come from plant food and animals that eat wild plant food.

Today, this balance has shifted to 10:1 or even 20:1! What this means is that we consume 10 (or 20) times more omega-6s than omega-3s.

Why this is a problem: Research has shown that too high of a ratio of omega-6 to omega-3s, can cause heart disease, along with a whole host of other illnesses. This is most likely because omega-6 has inflammatory properties, while omega-3 is anti-inflammatory. With the high dose of omega-6 that we consume, it is likely that most of us experience some sort of inflammation, the root of many health issues.

CALCIUM

Most people, no matter how nutritionally savvy, know that calcium helps builds strong bones and teeth. Calcium has other functions as well, such as maintaining healthy muscle tissue and supporting the healthy function of nerves and muscles—it even helps your blood to clot. Without enough calcium in your diet, your bones can grow brittle and you may experience frequent breaks and fractures; you may experience muscle aches, muscle spasms, and even that prickly tingly sensation in your hands or feet. In children, a deficiency of calcium can cause retarded growth or deformed skeletal formation.

Something else that everyone may not know: Plant foods, such as kale, can be terrific sources of well-digested, easily-absorbed calcium. (Yes, we're so used to seeing milk mustaches that it is hard to think of calcium coming from any source other than a cow!) One cup of cooked kale 93.60 mg of calcium, which is 9.4 percent of an adult's daily recommended amount.

CALCIUM: THE NAME

The word calcium is a geological one, coming from the Latin word *calx*, meaning limestone, a sedentary rock formed of calcite and aragonite, two forms of calcium carbonate crystals.

COPPER

Copper is the third most abundant trace mineral in the body; it's also responsible for helping enzymes function properly in our bodies. It also helps the body utilize iron, eliminate free radicals, create bone and connective tissue and produce the hair and skin pigment known as melanin.

Because it is found in most plant food and seafood, deficiency is rare, though lack of copper can lead to elevated LDL cholesterol levels, skin sores, anemia, susceptibility to infection, weakness, fatigue, osteoporosis, joint aches, shortness of breath, ruptured blood vessels, irregular heartbeat, and poor thyroid function. (An interesting bit of trivia: Many vegetables and whole grains grown today are lower in copper than they were during the mid-1900s and earlier, thanks to depletion of copper from the soil.) One cup of kale provides a respectable .20 mg of copper, which is 10 percent of an adult's daily recommended allowance of the mineral.

IRON

Iron is found in every cell of the body. One of its most high-profile functions is serving as the core of the hemoglobin molecule. This is the part of the red blood cell responsible for transporting life-sustaining oxygen throughout the body. Iron also helps the body utilize energy, utilize fat, and aids immune system function.

ABOUT COPPER POTS

Your body needs some copper to perform most body functions. Fortunately it's an easy mineral to get your fill of, as it's in a wide range of animal and plant foods, including grains and legumes. That said, there is such thing as too much copper, especially for those who use unlined copper cookware. The mineral leaches into food when copper pans are heated or come in contact with acidic ingredients, such as tomatoes or citrus. Signs of too much copper include vomiting, diarrhea, and nausea. If you're going to use copper cooking vessels, be safe and make sure they're lined with tin or another metal.

Dietary iron comes in two forms, heme iron (the kind in animal flesh) and non-heme iron (the type found in kale and other plant foods). A lot of attention is given to the two types of iron—which one is better? Which one does the body absorb more thoroughly? Which one does this, that, or the other? Here's the scoop: The body uses heme iron (again, the type from animal products) most efficiently, absorbing it at a rate of 7 to 35 percent depending upon the person. Non-heme iron (the kind from plant sources), normally gets absorbed at a rate of 2 to 20 percent. What this means is just because you eat a certain amount of iron—regardless of the source—doesn't mean your body is going to metabolize all of it.

Fortunately for your body—and your taste buds—kale contains iron! A one-cup serving of cooked kale contains 1.17 mg of iron, providing 6.5 percent of an adult's daily recommended amount of the mineral.

ARE YOU IRON DEFICIENT? JOIN THE CLUB.

The word anemia means "without blood." This refers to a deficiency in iron-rich red blood cells. Symptoms include fatigue, brain fog, memory loss, irritability, shortness of breath, dizziness, sallow skin, and blurry vision. Unfortunately, the disease is common, affecting an estimated 400 million women worldwide. In the United States alone, 20 percent of all women of childbearing age have iron deficiency anemia. Only 2 percent of men the same age experience anemia. Why the gender difference? Women menstruate, which means a regular and heavy loss of iron.

MANGANESE

Manganese is a trace mineral, which means the body needs it in very small amounts. It was first recognized as a nutrient in 1931 by researchers who were studying deficiency diseases in laboratory animals. It was found that animals with low levels of what we now call manganese suffered from weakness, retarded growth and infertility.

Manganese works as an enzyme activator. What this means is it activates the enzymes that are responsible for body functions. Without enough manganese, the body can exhibit a very large range of deficiency symptoms, including high blood sugar levels, diabetes, rashes, bone loss, abnormally low cholesterol levels, allergies, asthma, dizziness, hearing loss, learning disabilities, multiple sclerosis, premenstrual syndrome, rheumatoid arthritis, schizophrenia, infertility, nausea, vomiting, muscle weakness, vertigo, convulsions, recurring sprained muscles, paralysis, and/or blindness.

Fortunately, getting enough manganese isn't difficult. Kale is an excellent source of the mineral. One cup of the cooked greens contains .54 mcg, which is 27 percent of an adult's daily recommended allowance of manganese.

MANGANESE: DID YOU KNOW....?

The mineral manganese was found in a black mineral from the ancient Greek kingdom of Magnesia called *magnes*.

SIGNS OF MAGNESIUM DEFICIENCY

- Headaches
- Fatigue
- Sleep disturbances, insomnia
- Muscle weakness, tremors, or spasms
- Imbalanced blood sugar levels
- Elevated blood pressure
- Heart arrhythmia, irregular contraction, or increased heart rate
- Softening and weakening of bones

MAGNESIUM

Did you know that magnesium is the second most abundant mineral in your body? It's true! Human bodies contain about 25 grams of it, mostly in the skeleton. Furthermore, the mineral plays a role not only in the skeleton, but in every living cell in the human body. In fact, magnesium is involved in over 300 biochemical reactions in the body. Its presence is crucial to glucose and fat breakdown; reduction of proteins, enzymes and antioxidants such as glutathione; creation of DNA and RNA; and regulation of cholesterol production.

Magnesium is known as a macromineral, one that our food must provide. Kale, containing moderate amounts of this nutrient, can help you get the daily magnesium you need. One cup of the cooked greens provides 23.40 mg and 5.8 percent of an adult's daily recommended allowance of the mineral.

PHOSPHOROUS

Phosphorus is found in every cell in the body, concentrated most heavily in bones and teeth—perhaps it's not surprising that the mineral's primary function is in the formation of bone and teeth? Phosphorous also works with the B vitamins in nerve conduction and contraction of muscles; in addition, it helps maintain your heart's regular beat and healthy kidney function.

Because phosphorous is found in so many foods, deficiency is extremely rare. Animal products are the richest source of the mineral, but kale contains a moderate amount as well. One cup of cooked kale provides 36.40 mg and 3.6 percent of an adult's daily recommended allowance of phosphorous.

PHOSPHORUS: TOO MUCH OF A GOOD THING

Americans drink more soda—regular and diet—than any other people in the world. In fact, the average American drinks 170 liters of soda per year. To put things in perspective, the average citizen of France consumes 43 liters of soda per year, Italians drink 46 liters. Why this is a problem? Soda contributes to everything from obesity to diabetes to tooth decay. Soda is also high in phosphorus, which can lead to reduced bone density, osteoporosis, and cardiovascular disease. If you are drinking more than three servings of soda a week, cut down. For your health's sake.

TRYPTOPHAN: DID YOU KNOW...?

Tryptophan is an essential amino acid but also the least abundant, generally found in smaller quantities and in fewer number of foods than other amino acids.

TRYPTOPHAN

Tryptophan is one of the ten essential amino acids that the body uses to synthesize protein. But you may know the ingredient not for what it is, but what it does: No doubt you've heard the bit about Thanksgiving meals causing sleepiness because of the tryptophan in the turkey? Because of its calming effect on the nervous system and its role in helping the body fall asleep, tryptophan is often referred to as "the sleepy nutrient." Indeed, tryptophan is a precursor for serotonin, a neurotransmitter that helps the body regulate sleep, mood, and even appetite. Other tasks tryptophan attends to include helping treat headaches, easing premenstrual syndrome, and regulating weight by reducing those tough carb cravings.

One cup of kale contains .03 grams of tryptophan, which is 9.4 percent of an adult's daily allowance. This is enough of the mineral to contribute toward your body's requirement, but not enough to send you to sleep!

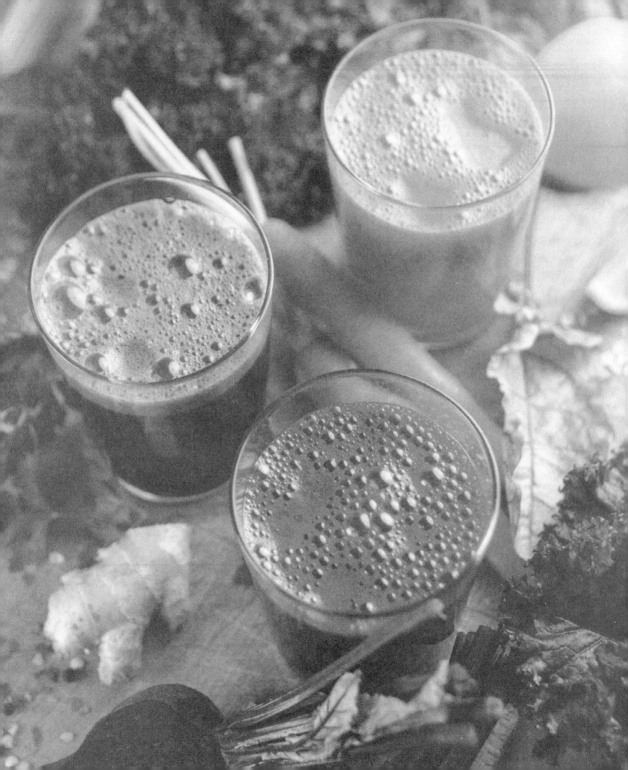

CHAPTER 3

DRINK YOUR KALE!

People come to kale in different ways. For many people, it's kale chips. Others are lured in by a raw kale salad. Still others grow up eating sautéed kale or kale soup. But a large portion of people in the "health set" first stumble upon kale as the secret ingredient in their health club's green drink or the neighborhood raw food joint's superfood smoothie.

This is a perfect way to be introduced to this easygoing, high-nutrient powerhouse. Blending kale into a drink makes it easy to create your own health bar-style beverages at home. But before you start, let's talk blenders. If you've got a turbocharged VitaMix or BlendTec (the gold standards of the health food world), go ahead and use any type of kale you'd like. Your blender is so powerful, you could even use the leaf's rib.

Everyone else will want to stick to the more tender baby kale leaves. They break down more easily and thoroughly than their mature counterparts, which is important when using a mainstream kitchen blender.

If you've got a juicer, you'll find plenty of recipes here to get you started. And yes, you can use whatever type of kale you'd like—with the rib.

Lastly, a health warning: If you have suffered from a kidney stone or have been told to take it easy on foods with oxalic acid, ask your health care professional about drinking smoothies and juices containing raw kale. As you learned in Chapter Two, raw kale contains oxalic acid, which can contribute to kidney stone formation in some people.

If you're told to hold off on raw kale recipes, we've got you covered. There are plenty of cooked kale recipes throughout this book to enjoy. If you've got your heart set on a kale drink, however, here's something to try: Follow any of the blender recipes below (this trick won't work for juicer drinks) and where raw kale is listed, simply swap in ¼ to ⅓ cup of cooked unseasoned kale. Easy! Start your blenders!

SHAKES

CHOCO-KALE HEALTH SHAKE

MAKES 1 TO 2 SERVINGS

This yummy shake combines chocolate, coconut, and kale to create a sweet source of nutrients and healthy fats. If you're giving it to kids or picky adults, leave out the spirulina and chlorophyll, which can give a subtle yet decidedly "green" taste to the drink.

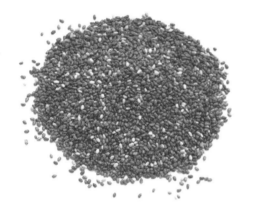

1   tablespoon chia seed
2   or 3 tablespoons raw cacao powder or ¼ cup carob or cacao nibs
2   cups coconut milk
2   cups raw baby kale (mature kale is just too "kaley" for this)
½   avocado
1   teaspoon cinnamon
8   ice cubes
    Stevia to taste

CACAO VS. COCOA

Cacao (pronounced cah-COW) is made of the solids left behind after the liquid (called "liquor" or "liqueur") and butter have been removed from the cacao beans. There is loud, frequent debate among foodies about the difference between cacao and cocoa powders. In truth, there is no difference, other than spelling. If you come across the word "raw" tacked onto cacao powder, it simply means that the product has not been heated above 110°F.

Optional: 1 or 2 tablespoons virgin organic coconut oil
Optional: 1 scoop chocolate or vanilla flavor protein powder (rice, hemp, legume, whey, etc.)
Optional: ¼ to ½ teaspoon spirulina or chlorophyll powder

1. Add all ingredients to a blender and liquefy using the most powerful setting. Blend until smooth.
2. Drink immediately.

MINT DESSERT SHAKE

MAKES 2 SERVINGS

Sometimes you want something creamy, sweet, and treat-like. But for whatever reason you also want this sweet thing to have some nutritional value. In my house, this is the recipe for

AVOCADOS—THE SEXIEST SUPERFOOD

Smooth and lush, with a rich texture, avocados are the darlings of the culinary world. But did you know that they are also bursting with a wide range of health-boosting benefits? Here are just a few of the reasons you should make avocados part of your weekly diet:

- Avocados are a powerful anti-inflammatory food, boasting a range of phytosterols, carotenoids, antioxidants, omega-3 fatty acids, and polyhydrozylated fatty acids, all of which help prevent or lessen arthritis joint afflictions, cardiovascular disease, and auto-immune disease.
- Avocados help the body absorb other nutrients. For instance, one cup of fresh avocado, when eaten with a salad or other food, can increase the body's absorption of carotenoids from that food between 200 to 400 percent.
- One cup of avocado supplies 30 percent of the daily recommendation of fiber.
- Avocado has been found to help prevent the occurrence of cancers of the mouth, skin, and prostate gland, probably due to its antioxidant boosting ability and its high content of anti-inflammatory nutrients.
- One cup of avocado has over 35 percent of one's daily allowance for vitamin K, a vitamin associated with bone formation and proper blood clotting, as well as the transport of calcium through the body.
- Individuals with latex allergies should eat limit their avocado consumption or avoid it completely. Unfortunately, the fruit contains high amounts of something called chitinase enzymes, which are associated with latex allergies. Cooking the food lightly does slightly deactivate these enzymes.

those times. It's our birthday go-to, celebrating a straight-A report card go-to, and even where we turn when we need to drown our sorrows. We use coconut-based ice cream and milk, but you can use whatever milk you love, including rice, hemp, hazelnut, oat, almond, goat, or cow.

2   to 3 cups milk (depending on how thick you like your shake) of your choice (we use coconut)

2   cups vanilla or mint-chocolate chip ice cream (we use coconut)

1   cup baby kale leaves

¼   to ½ avocado

2   drops peppermint extract

1. Put all ingredients into a blender and blend until kale has been liquidized and all ingredients have been blended.

NUTTY CHOCO-KALE SHAKE

MAKES 1 TO 2 SERVINGS

If you tolerate nuts well, they make a high-protein, high-fiber, high-nutrient addition to the smoothies. You can make it easy on yourself and throw a handful of nuts into any smoothie you are making or spoon in a dollop of nut butter. Or, you can try this yummy recipe. It is super satisfying and one of my kids' favorite after-homework treats.

2 *cups non-dairy milk of choice*
1 *cup baby kale leaves*
¼ *cup nut butter of choice*
2 *tablespoons honey, agave or maple syrup*
2 *tablespoons cocoa*
Optional: 1 banana

1. Put all ingredients into a blender and blend until kale has been liquidized and all ingredients have been blended.

SMOOTHIES

KALE BERRY BLAST

MAKES 1 SERVING

Kale, strawberries, and blueberries—three potent superfoods, all brimming with vitamins and antioxidants. To keep natural sugar intake at a minimum, I prefer to use water to make this.

1½ *cup water, coconut water, or fruit juice of choice*
½ *cup fresh or frozen blueberries*
½ *cup fresh or frozen strawberries*
1 *cup baby kale leaves*

1. Put all ingredients into a blender and blend until kale has been liquidized and all ingredients have been blended.

CREAMY KALE SMOOTHIE

MAKES 1 SERVING

This mild-tasting, creamy smoothie is a great introduction to green drinks. It's one of my kids' absolute favorites. For more sweetness, blend in a peeled banana or pear.

1½ cup unsweetened almond, hazelnut, coconut, rice, or hemp milk
1 cup baby kale
¼ cup raw cashews (you can also use almonds or walnuts)
½ avocado
Optional: A splash of vanilla or almond extract

1. Put all ingredients into a blender and blend until kale has been liquidized and all ingredients have been blended.

CASHEW TRIVIA

Lower in fat than other nuts, high in protein, and addictively delicious, cashews are the darlings of the snack world. You know you love them, but did you know this about them?

- Cashews are native to the coastal regions of Brazil.
- The cashew nut is actually the kidney-shaped seed that sits at the bottom of the cashew apple, a delicacy in Brazil and the Caribbean, where the fruit grows prolifically.
- Cashews are always sold shelled. Why? Because the interior of the cashew shell contains a caustic resin known as cashew balm, which is carefully removed before nuts are packaged for human consumption. This resin is used to make insecticides and varnishes.
- Cashew's scientific name is Anacardium occidentale.
- Cashews belong to the same family as the pistachio and mango.
- In the 16th century, Portuguese explorers took cashew trees from Brazil and introduced them to other tropical countries, including India and Africa.
- Currently, the leading commercial providers of cashews are Brazil, Mozambique, Tanzania, and Nigeria.
- Cashew wood is a precious, much-prized resource in Brazil.

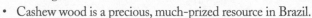

THE BEST SMOOTHIES

A smoothie is a blended drink containing healthy ingredients (think milkshake without the dairy and ice cream!). Really, you can blend any fruit or veggie together and get a smoothie—the recipes in this section are simply some of our favorites. Before you begin, however, these tips can make your smoothie-making adventures to be even more successful:

- If your smoothie is too thick, add more water or juice or other liquid.
- Process your smoothie for as long as you need to in order to get a smooth, silky drink. No one wants to be drinking bits of pulp.
- If you're using a weaker blender, you may find it necessary to pour the liquid through a colander or strainer to remove large bits of fiber.
- Kale and other greens can often create a green foam when whirred in a blender or when juiced. This foam is edible and healthy—however (total honesty here!) most people loathe the stuff. My own kids call it pond scum. That's why we always take a spatula and scrape it off into the sink or into a compost pile.

KALE LIME SLUSHY

MAKES 4 SERVINGS

This icy cold treat is a summer staple in our house. It is refreshing, fun, tangy, and (yep!) healthy! Everything you could want from a slushy!

1   *cup baby kale leaves*
½   *cup applesauce or pearsauce*
2   *cups water or coconut water*
1   *can limeade (or lemonade) concentrate,*
    preferably organic
8   *to 10 ice cubes*

1. Put all ingredients except ice into a blender and blend until kale has been liquidized.

2. Add limeade concentrate and ice to blender and pulse until drink is icy and well-blended.

BANANA KALE SMOOTHIE

MAKES 1 SERVING

If you've ever picked up one of those bottled green drinks, you know how sweet and thick they are. Banana is the reason why. It provides intense sweetness and a thick creamy quality to non-dairy smoothies, like this one. For a creamier smoothie, use coconut milk for the liquid.

1   *medium banana, ripe*
1   *cup baby leaf kale*
1½ *cup water, coconut water,t or fruit juice of choice*
    Squirt lemon juice
Optional: 1 slice fresh ginger

1. Put all ingredients into a blender and blend until kale has been liquidized and all ingredients have been blended.

GO BANANAS

Ah, the banana! This ubiquitous yellow fruit is strongly associated in the U.S. with breakfast, but how well do you really know this tropical treat? Read on:

- A banana plant grows between 10 to 26 feet.
- Banana plants belong to the same family as the lily and the orchid.
- Bananas grow in clusters of 50–150 fruits known as "hands."
- A medium-size banana contains 467 mg of potassium and only 1 mg of sodium.
- Most of today's bananas are grown in tropical and subtropical countries, most commonly Costa Rica and Ecuador, but also Mexico and Brazil.
- In addition to its cardiovascular benefits, the potassium found in bananas may also help to promote bone health. Potassium may counteract the increased urinary calcium loss caused by the high-salt diets typical of most Americans, thus helping to prevent bones from thinning out at a fast rate.
- Bananas have long been recognized for their antacid effects that protect against stomach ulcers and ulcer damage. In an animal study, researchers found that fresh bananas protected the animals' stomachs from wounds.
- Because they are high in electrolytes, bananas are a traditional cure for diarrhea.
- Bananas contain high levels of a compound called fructooligosaccharide. This probiotic nourishes beneficial bacteria in the colon, improving the body's ability to absorb nutrients. This, in turn, decreases the body's risk of colon cancer.
- It's not known exactly where bananas originated, though many experts believe the fruit was first grown in Malaysia around 4,000 years ago. From there, they spread throughout the Philippines and then India, where they were first encountered by Alexander the Great's soldiers in 3227 BCE.
- Bananas spread first to the Middle East, then Africa, where they were discovered by Portuguese explorers on their way to the New World. They were widely planted in what is now South and Central America.
- Bananas were not brought to the United States until late in the 19th century. Because they were so fragile, bananas were at first only available in the sea towns where they were unloaded.

STEPHANIE'S BUILD-YOUR-OWN KALE SMOOTHIE BLUEPRINT

MAKES 1 TO 2 SERVINGS

This is the blueprint I give to my private clients, my detox clients, and my weight loss clients. It's a fun mix-and-match blueprint that allows you to make a different smoothie every day if you'd like, depending upon what you have available in our kitchen and what you feel like. You can even tailor it to suit specific health needs.

2 *cups liquid of choice (I use a mixture of water and coconut water or just regular water.) Add more water if you want the drink more "liquidy"*

1 *cucumber, peeled and cut into large chunks so your blender can process it better*

1 *to 2 cups baby kale, spinach or salad greens*

3 *or 4 sprigs parsley or mint*

Optional: Squirt of lemon or lime—fantastic for helping to flush toxins from the body

Optional: 1 tablespoon coconut oil and/or ½ of an avocado and/or 2 tablespoons nut butter and/or ¼ cup nuts of choice. (These are all fantastic sources of brain-nourishing, cardiovascular-helping fats)

Optional: 1 teaspoon spirulina powder and/or 1 teaspoon greens powder, and/or 1 to 2 tablespoons chia seed, and/or 1 tablespoon rice or legume-based protein powder.

Optional: 1 or 2 tablespoons maple syrup, honey, or agave

1. Fill your blender with your chosen liquid and ingredients. Process as long as necessary to create a smooth drink.

THE MARVELS OF MAPLE

Maple syrup is the sweet sap of the sugar, black, and red maple trees, and it's a terrific sweetener to add to the health-supportive kitchen. That's because, ounce for ounce, maple contains less calories and more minerals than honey or sugar. Look for grade B or Dark Amber grade maple—it's darker and richer in taste than the lighter, less complex Grade A or Light Amber. All shades, however, are high in manganese and zinc, two minerals essential for health immune system function.

SUPERFOOD PROTEIN SMOOTHIE

MAKES 1 TO 2 SERVINGS

This fun smoothie is packed with all kinds of superfoods. It's as perfect for someone training for a marathon as it is for anyone convalescing from an illness. It's tasty, too!

1½ *cups coconut water*

1 *cup baby kale leaf*

2 *tablespoons coconut oil*

1 *tablespoon maple, honey, or agave*

¼ *cup raw walnuts*

¼ *cup raw cashews*

2 *tablespoons chia*

2 *tablespoons goji berries*

1 *slice ginger (as big or small as you'd like)*

1. Put all ingredients into a blender and blend until kale has been liquidized and all ingredients have been blended.

EASY ENERGY

Chia has been used for energy since BCE times. Aztec warriors and athletes were thought to have performed on as little as one tablespoon of chia per day. The seeds are about 20 percent protein per weight and offer about 2 grams of protein per tablespoon. This makes chia ideal for increasing the protein content in any low-protein food. In fact, Aztec warriors and runners are believed to have sustained themselves for an entire day on just a tablespoon of chia, making it one of the original "breakfasts of champions." Further, chia also helps the body maintain sustained hydration, which can come in handy for anyone engaged in heavy, prolonged activity.

TROPICAL SMOOTHIE
MAKES 1 SERVING

Sweet and soothing, this fruity smoothie is loved by everyone. Kids love it when it's made with pineapple juice. Thanks to the mango, the drink is especially high in vitamin A, which is important for healthy eyesight and skin, and immune system function.

1½ cup water, coconut water, or pineapple juice (you can use a combination of these)
1   cup frozen mango chunks
½   cup baby kale
     Squirt or two of lemon or lime juice

1. Put all ingredients into a blender and blend until kale has been liquidized and all ingredients have been blended.

MANGO MADNESS!

Sweet, soft, and sensual, mangos are one of my favorite tropical fruits. Just as wonderful as their full-bodied flavor? Mangos are also loaded with health benefits:
- One average size mango contains 105 calories and provides 76 percent of an adult's daily requirement of vitamin C, 25 percent vitamin A, and 11 percent vitamin B6.
- Mangos provide insoluble fiber, which helps promote digestive health.
- Research has shown that the antioxidant compounds in mango help protect against colon, breast, leukemia, and prostate cancers. These compounds include quercetin, isoquercitrin, astragalin, fisetin, gallic acid, and methylgallat.
- The high levels of fiber, pectin and vitamin C help to lower serum cholesterol levels.
- Vitamins C and vitamin A in mangos, plus 25 different kinds of carotenoids, keep the immune system healthy and strong.

SMOOTHIES ON THE ROAD

Smoothies are a fantastic way to give yourself a concentrated dose of super-nutrients in one sitting. They can even be made on the road—in fact, they are ideal for busy types who like to start their days off in a powerful way. To ensure you are set-up for success while you're on the road, follow these easy tips.

- Carry a small portable blender—such as a Magic Bullet—in your handbag or luggage, while you're traveling.
- Opt for pre-washed baby kale, baby spinach, or baby salad greens—they break down much easier in a small, portable blender. Save the heavy greens for a hardcore blender.
- For liquid, use water from the tap, or pack a few aseptic single-serving size containers of coconut water or other beverages.

JUICE

KALE JUICE STRAIGHT UP

Kale juice is one of the most nutritious juices around. It boasts extremely powerful antioxidant, anti-inflammatory, and anti-cancer properties. It strengthens the immune system and is loaded with beta carotene, vitamin C, vitamin K, lutein, zeaxanthin, and calcium. It's also pretty hard to stomach on its own. Of course you can try, but you may find it to be so "green-tasting" (as one of my sons says), that you just cannot stand it. (I'm just being honest!) That's why I've collected a few blended juice recipes, which will allow you to enjoy the enormous benefits kale juice has to offer, in a more palatable format. Enjoy!

TO DILUTE OR NOT TO DILUTE? THAT IS THE QUESTION!

Many people dilute their fresh-pressed juice with pure water. This is an easy way to lighten up heavy juices (think those made solely of root veggies) or give strong-tasting juices a milder taste. Where do I fall on the dilution question? Nowhere, really. If I make a juice with lots of beets or carrots (or other root vegetables), I almost always add a half cup to two cups of water. I'll also add one or two cups of water if it looks like the juice I made isn't going to stretch far enough to serve four people (myself, Leif, Anders, and Axel—my poor husband won't go near juice!). I typically do not dilute juice when it contains a lot of watery fruits and vegetables, such as cucumber or citrus. In other words, there is no hard-and-fast dilution rule. It's all good.

LOSE THE BLOAT KALE DRINK

MAKES 1 SERVING

This is the juice I sip when I wake up retaining water or have a black-tie event and for some reason, can't comfortably fit into my dress. It is a diuretic and helps safely (yet quickly!) flush excess water from the body. (Just a warning: The dandelion gives this drink a bitter flavor, a flavor I happen to like. Feel free to add a cup of pineapple to the mix if you'd like.)

5 *kale leaves*
1 *medium to large cucumber, cut into slices small enough to fit in your juicer's feed tube*
2 *celery stalks*
10 *dandelion leaves*
10 *sprigs parsley*
   1-inch ginger
1 *lemon*

1. Run all ingredients through the juicer's feed tube. Strain finished liquid if necessary.

PARSLEY POWER

If you haven't yet juiced or blended parsley into one of your drinks, I have one question: What are you waiting for? This refreshing herb is more nutrient-dense than many vegetables.

- Parsley's volatile oils have been shown to inhibit tumor formation in animal studies, and particularly, tumor formation in the lungs.
- Two tablespoons of parsley provide 155.8% of the body's requirement of vitamin K, 16.8% of vitamin C, and 12.8% of vitamin A.
- Parsley is native to Mediterranean Europe.
- Parsley, which has been grown domestically for more than 2,000 years, was originally used not as a food, but as a medicine.
- The Greeks considered parsley to be sacred and used it for decorating tombs and celebrating winning athletes.
- Parsley contains strong antioxidants called flavonoids, which strengthen the body's immune system.

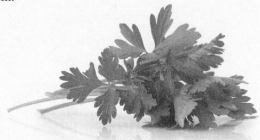

RED KALE JUICE

MAKES 2 OR MORE SERVINGS

For this drink I specify red kale. Yes, you can use other varieties, but the juice's color won't be as pretty. It'll still taste great and be full of antioxidants. I begin making this drink around Thanksgiving when cranberries appear in stores.

5 *leaves red kale*
1 *cup fresh cranberries*
2 *medium beets, cut into slices small enough to fit in your juicer's feed tube*
   ½-inch piece of ginger
1 *blood orange, peeled and sectioned*

1. Run all ingredients through the juicer's feed tube. Strain finished liquid if necessary.

REFRESHING KALE COOLER

MAKES 4 OR MORE SERVINGS

This fun recipe requires you to add something to the juice after pressing it. It's a great warm-weather drink, beloved by even the most ardent kale haters.

1 *medium to large cucumber, cut into sections small enough to fit in your juicer's feed tube*
1 *bunch kale*
3 *apples, cut into slices small enough to fit in our juicer's feed tube*
1 *lemon or lime, cut into slices small enough to fit in your juicer's feed tube*
   1-inch section of ginger
1 *to 2 cups coconut water*

1. Run all ingredients through the juicer's feed tube. Strain finished liquid if necessary.
2. Add 1 to 2 cups of coconut water to the pressed juice. Stir to combine. Drink immediately.

STAY-WELL KALE JUICE
MAKES 2 OR MORE SERVINGS

This is the juice I make for my kids when a cold is going through their school. It is rich in enzymes and antioxidants. It also tastes good.

1   *cup pineapple, cut into sections small enough to fit in your juicer's feed tube*
1   *bunch kale*
2   *large cucumbers, cut into sections small enough to fit in your juicer's feed tube*
1   *lemon, cut into sections small enough to fit in your juicer's feed tube*
¼   *cup mint*
    ½-inch slice ginger

1. Run all ingredients through the juicer's feed tube. Strain finished liquid if necessary.

WHY YOU NEED PINEAPPLE

When I was growing up, one of the moms on our street would always juice a pineapple for me anytime I caught a cold. "It's the enzymes," she'd say knowingly. "They eat away the virus." And it did seem as though the cold would lessen after downing that sweet, tangy juice. Time passed and I grew up. Without even questioning, I also juice a pineapple anytime one of my children, my husband, or I come down with a cold. After studying nutrition, I learned that the pineapple's enzymes are anti-inflammatory and certainly work to keep you healthy, but it was probably the fruit's high vitamin C content (75 percent of the daily recommended allowance) at work in wiping out offending viruses.

MUCH TO-DO ABOUT JUICERS

There's a lot of debate in the juicing world around juicer types, and which type makes the best, healthiest juice. Twin-gear or triturating juicers flatten produce between two rollers. They work excruciatingly slow, but because they do not generate any heat, it's believed that the juice's nutrient profile stays most intact. Masticating juicers (I've got one of these) "chew" the produce sending the juice down one tube and the pulp down another. These do warm up produce slightly, but are considered the most healthful and effective juicers for home use. Centrifugal juicers are the fastest and easiest to clean of the bunch, and are also the most economical. They work by grating the fruit or vegetable into a pulp, and then use centrifugal force to push the pulp against a strainer screen by spinning it at a very high RPM. The juice is forced from the screen and down a juice shoot. While centrifugal juicers do cause the most "damage" to nutrients, fresh-pressed juice made with them is still a deeply nourishing food. My take: Use whatever juicer you like enough to operate on a daily basis! Fresh kale juice does the most good when consumed daily.

SUNSHINE JUICE

MAKES 2 OR MORE SERVINGS

Give my second son, Anders, a collection of grapefruits, oranges, lemons, limes, oranges, pomelos, and tangerines and he is in heaven. He is definitely my citrus kid. Not surprisingly, this juice is his favorite. If, like Anders and me, you love bitter flavors, add a grapefruit to the mix.

5   *kale leaves*

1   *apple, cut into slices small enough to fit in your juicer's feed tube*

1   *orange, peeled and sectioned*

1   *tangerine or Clementine, peeled and sectioned*

½   *lemon*

½   *lime*

1. Run all ingredients through the juicer's feed tube. Strain finished liquid if necessary.

SUGAR? CHECK THE INDEX!

If you're health conscious, you've probably heard the term "glycemic index." This list of common foods shows which ingredients are best at creating stable blood sugar and which wreck havoc, creating dramatic spikes then falls in blood glucose levels (leaving you feeling tired, irritable, with insatiable cravings). For ideal health, you want to choose foods that are low on the glycemic index—closer to a "1"—and avoid those foods which are rated higher (the highest of them rate around 100). Here's a list of popular smoothie and juice ingredients and where they stand on the glycemic index, from highest to lowest:

Watermelon	72	Grapefruit	25
Cherries	63	Raspberries	2
Banana, ripe	62	Broccoli	0
Grapes	59	Celery	0
Blueberries	53	Cucumber	0
Apple juice, unsweetened	44	Ginger	0
Dates, dried	42	Green beans	0
Peach	42	Kale	0
Carrots	41	Lemons	0
Orange	40	Lettuce	0
Strawberries	40	Limes	0
Apple	39	Spinach	0
Pear	38	Tomatoes	0
Prunes	29	Zucchini	0

V8-STYLE JUICE

MAKES 4 OR MORE SERVINGS

My four-year-old son, Axel, is crazy for commercial tomato and V8-style juices. Up until recently I always bought several cans and bottles of the stuff each week. However, when a client gave me a shopping bag of tomatoes, I decided to make my own tomato-veggie blend. Axel loves it just as much as the stuff from a can! (I do, too.)

3   *large tomatoes, cut into slices small enough*
    to fit in your juicer's feed tube (feel free to
    use more tomatoes if you're lucky enough
    to have a surplus)
½   *bunch kale, washed and dried*
1   *celery stalk*
1   *small to medium cucumber*
1   *carrot*
2   *to 4 sprigs of parsley, stem included*
½   *red or green bell pepper*
1   *half lemon*
1   *small garlic clove*
Optional: 1 sliver fresh jalapeño pepper
    or a radish
Optional: A shake of Tabasco sauce for
    finished juice

1. Run all ingredients through the juicer's feed tube. Strain finished liquid if necessary. Season with Tabasco sauce if desired.

SERIOUSLY? GARLIC JUICE?

I know you've already heard what a powerful ingredient garlic is. It supercharges the immune system to fight off marauding viruses, fungi and bacteria. It helps with high blood pressure and cholesterol. Garlic has also been shown to help the body heal faster and more thoroughly. But juicing it? Adding it to smoothies?

Yes, I am serious. I really am. You may not want to add a clove of garlic to your sweet berry supreme smoothie, but it's the perfect addition to any tomato-based drinks or veggie-heavy green juices. Just one clove is all you need in order to get all those juicy benefits. Just one clove. Try it! (I dare you.)

TOMATO TALES

In many parts of the world—think North America and Europe—nothing says summer like "tomato." This sunny vegetable (botanically a fruit) is as loved for its addictive taste as its powerful nutrient profile: vitamins A, B-complex, and C, antioxidants, potassium, and phosphorous. But in some dietary systems (such as macrobiotics), tomatoes are forbidden as a weakening food that ruins the gastrointestinal tract. Other healing systems, such as Ayurveda, applaud tomatoes when cooked with a generous amount of warming cumin and turmeric. My advice: If raw tomatoes bother you, try them cooked. If you can eat tomatoes with impunity, toss one into the juicer to make your own yummy V8-style drink.

WARMING AUTUMN KALE JUICE

MAKES 2 OR MORE SERVINGS

I generally try not to mix green veggies with orange or red veggies when I juice. This has nothing to do with health and everything to do with aesthetics: In my house we enjoy our juice out of glass tumblers and when I mix green and orange and red, what I get is an unattractive gray-brown color, which my junior high school art teacher called "taupe." Not something the kids want to consume. This recipe is an exception. I love the sweet, deep flavor that comes when I juice carrots and beets. Plus, this recipe is a powerful one, great for detoxing, fantastic for the skin, and superb for the immune system.

1   *bunch kale*
2   *large beets or medium sweet potatoes, cut into slices small enough to fit in your juicer's feed tube*
4   *large carrots, cut into slices small enough to fit in your juicer's feed tube*
2   *large apple or 3 pears, cut into slices small enough to fit in your juicer's feed tube*
½   *to 1 lemon, cut into slices small enough to fit in your juicer's feed tube*

1. Run all ingredients through the juicer's feed tube. Strain finished liquid if necessary.

WHAT IS AN ANTIOXIDANT?

To understand antioxidants, it's important to first understand oxidants. Oxidation is a chemical reaction that transfers electrons or hydrogen from a substance to an oxidizing agent. Oxidation reactions can produce free radicals, or oxidants. In turn, these radicals can start chain reactions. When the chain reaction occurs in a cell, it can cause damage or death to the cell. An antioxidant is a molecule capable of inhibiting the oxidation of other molecules.

The easiest place to get these protective molecules is from food. Namely, plant food. Brightly and darkly colored fruits and vegetables are some of the best sources of these powerful nutrients. Eating numerous servings of antioxidant-heavy food daily is one of the most effective ways to maintain wellness.

DRINK IMMEDIATELY!

You may have heard that fresh-pressed juice is most healthful if you can drink it immediately. Here's why: Immediately after being made, fruit and vegetable juice contains the highest levels of enzymes. The longer juice sits, the greater its exposure to oxygen. The longer it's exposed to oxygen, the more of its enzymes are affected by oxidation. After 20 minutes of exposure, the majority of enzymes in juice have been destroyed.

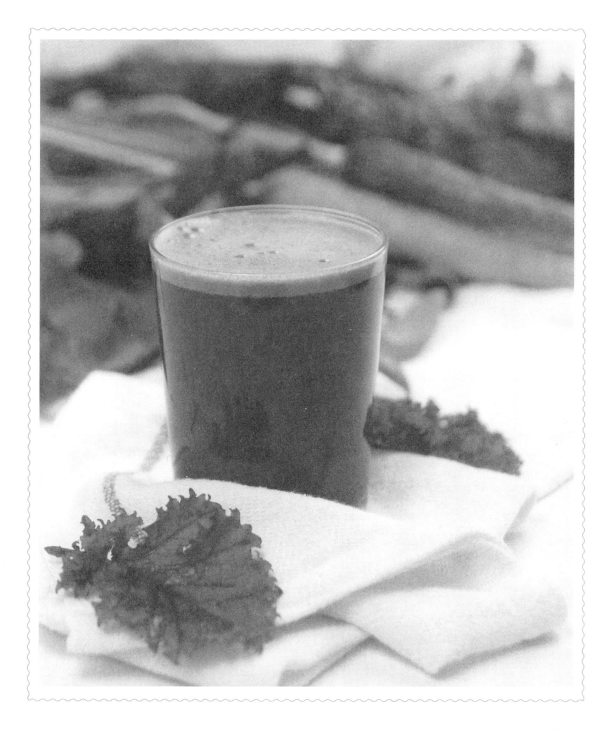

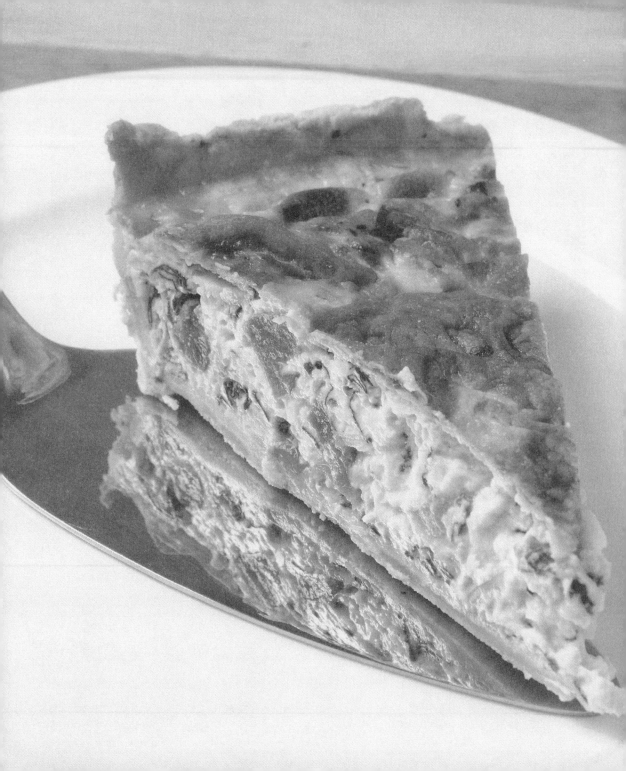

CHAPTER 4

BREAKFAST: START YOUR DAY WITH KALE

Kale for breakfast? I guess it does sound a bit strange, especially for those of you who grew up eating white-flour-and-dairy for breakfast. But consider this: In many parts of the world, veggies for breakfast are the norm. In places like India, China, Japan, Israel, Australia (with their ever-present broiled tomatoes), and Europe, people enjoy soup, raw veggies, veggie rice dishes, and more as their first meal of the day.

The trend is catching on in North America, especially with "health foodies" who wouldn't dream of starting their day without a green juice or smoothie. (If you're intrigued, turn to Chapter 3 for some of our favorite green drinks—all of which are awesome for breakfast.) But kale is so much more versatile than just beverages.

Kale pairs beautifully with a number of the foods you're already eating for breakfast. Check out these recipes to see what I mean.

EGGS

BREAKFAST CASSEROLE

MAKES 6 TO 8 SERVINGS

This is one of those simple, fast, filling, delicious dishes you see on brunch tables. In Australia, these are called "bakes." In the States, they're known as breakfast casseroles. Not that your guests care what you call this slightly exotic taste dish—they'll just want to dig in!

3 *tablespoons extra virgin olive oil*
¼ *teaspoon minced fresh ginger*
3 *large onions, chopped*
3 *cloves garlic, minced*
1 *teaspoon ground turmeric*
1½ *cup cooked, steamed or blanched kale, squeezed dry and coarsely chopped*
   Salt and pepper to taste
4 *tablespoons all-purpose flour or all-purpose gluten-free flour*
½ *teaspoon baking soda*
7 *eggs, beaten*
Optional: 2 tablespoons chopped parsley
Optional: paprika for garnish

1. Heat oven to 400°F.

2. Heat 2 tablespoons of the olive oil in a large skillet over medium-high heat. Add the ginger, onions, and garlic. Cook until soft, about 6 to 8 minutes.

3. Add turmeric and kale to the skillet, seasoning with salt and pepper as desired. Cook until tender, about 10 minutes.

4. Turn off the heat and stir in 3 tablespoons flour and the baking soda.

5. Stir eggs into kale mixture.

6. Prepare a 9- by 13-inch casserole dish by greasing with remaining tablespoon of olive oil and dusting with remaining two tablespoons of flour.

7. Pour egg-kale mixture into prepared pan and place in oven. Bake until set, about 25 to 30 minutes. (You do not want to overcook; the dish will be a bit wobbly in the middle.)

8. Optional: Garnish with chopped parsley and/or paprika.

ONIONS: NOTHING TO CRY OVER

Onions make everything taste better. A quick sauté in butter or oil does wonders for fried foods, a few slices of crisp onion makes any sandwich or burger taste better, and what is a soup, stew, braise or piece or roasted meat without onion? In addition to being de rigueur in any food-lover's kitchen, onions are also incredibly healthy. Consider:

- Onions have just 40 calories per 100 grams.
- Onions are rich in soluble dietary fiber.
- The compound allicin found in onions give them cancer-fighting properties. Allicin has also been found to have anti-bacterial, anti-viral, and antifungal activities.
- Onions help decrease the risk of coronary artery disease, stroke, and peripheral vascular diseases. Again, it's the allicin, which decreases blood vessel stiffness and reduces total blood pressure. It also blocks the formation of blood clots.
- Onions contain chromium, a trace mineral that helps insulin act on and control sugar levels in diabetes.
- They are also a good source of the antioxidant flavonoid quercetin, which is found to have anti-carcinogenic, anti-inflammatory, and anti-diabetic functions.
- Onions help strengthen and protect the immune system, thanks to high levels of the antioxidant, vitamin C.
- Manganese is found in onions. This mineral is required for normal growth and health. It helps your body break down fats, carbohydrates, and proteins.
- Onions are also rich in the B-complex group of vitamins, which help to maintain healthy skin and muscle and nervous system function.

KALE-BACON QUICHE CUPS

MAKES 6 SERVINGS

Kids love these, adults love these, frou-frou types like these! Easy to make, freezable, and fun to eat—you'll love them, too. Oh, and they contain kale!

8 eggs
2 tablespoons half and half or non-dairy cream
2 strips thick-cut bacon
1 cup chopped red bell pepper
¼ cup cooked, steamed, or blanched kale,
   coarsely chopped
2 to 3 green onions, chopped
⅛ to ¼ teaspoon sea salt
   Pinch red pepper flakes
   Pinch sweet paprika

1. Preheat oven to 350°F.
2. Grease the cups of a standard muffin tin.
3. Heat a medium skillet over medium high heat and add the chopped bacon. Sauté for 5 to 10 minutes until brown and crispy. Remove from pan and pat dry of grease.
4. Drain the bacon grease from the skillet to a heat-proof bowl. Reserve.
5. Add 1 tablespoon reserved bacon grease to the skillet. Sauté bell pepper and onion for 3 to 5 minutes, until soft.
6. Turn off heat and stir cooked kale into red pepper mixture.
7. In a medium bowl whisk together the eggs, salt, and half and half.
8. To the egg mixture, add the bacon and vegetable mixture, stirring until combined.
9. Pour the egg mixture into the muffin wells/sauté pan. (You may want to pour egg mixture from a large liquid measuring cup with a spout.) Top with Parmesan cheese and bake for 20 minutes or until just firm with browned edges.

BELLS OF THE VEGGIE BALL

Bell peppers—so named because of their blocky shape—are a veggie garden favorite. What you may not know, however, is that bell peppers aren't actually veggies. They're fruits, which boast over 195 percent of a body's daily requirement for vitamin C, 57 percent of vitamin A, and dozens of different carotenes and flavonoids, two families of antioxidants that help ward off cancers, viruses, bacteria, and fungi, as well as strengthen the immune system. Also known as capsicums (especially in England and Australia), these range in color from green to red in varying stages of ripeness. There are also brown, purple, yellow, orange, and black varieties.

KALE-MUSHROOM-POBLANO FRITTATA

MAKES 4 SERVINGS

If you're like me, you adore anything with a bit of bite to it, hence this delicious and hearty frittata. Use any type of mushrooms you'd like and when you're ready to branch out, experiment with other types of chili peppers. Notice the refreshing addition of cilantro. If you're a cilantro-hater, feel free to substitute chives or parsley. You'll need an ovenproof skillet for this one.

3 tablespoons extra-virgin olive oil
8 ounces assorted mushrooms (such as button, baby bella, crimini, oyster, and stemmed shiitake), thinly sliced
1 large fresh poblano chili, stemmed, seeded, thinly sliced into strips
1 cup chopped scallions
1 cup cooked, steamed, or blanched kale, squeezed dry and coarsely chopped
   Salt and freshly ground black pepper, to taste
6 large eggs
2 tablespoons chopped fresh cilantro
½ teaspoon ground cumin
Optional: Salsa for garnish

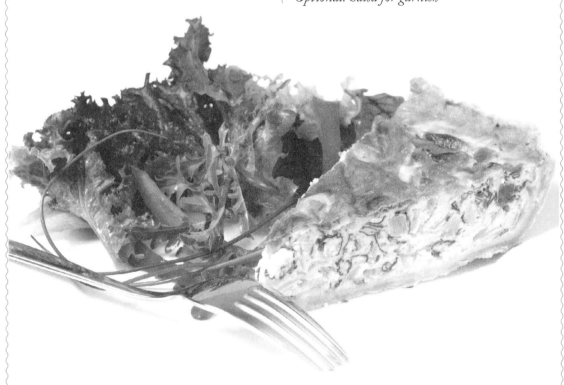

GOURMET SUPER VEGGIE!

In the current stampede to get more and more colorful veggies into our diets, it's easy to overlook the humble (and very uncolorful) mushroom. This is a darn shame, when you consider that mushrooms are not only exquisite-tasting, but antioxidant superpowers. They contain:

- B-complex vitamins, which play an important role in nervous system function.
- Riboflavin, to help maintain healthy red blood cells.
- Niacin, which ensures the digestive and nervous systems function properly.
- Selenium, a mineral that works as an antioxidant to protect body cells from damage that might lead to heart disease, some cancers, and other diseases of aging.
- Ergothioneine, a naturally occurring antioxidant that helps protect the body's cells.
- Copper, which helps make red blood cells, which in turn carry oxygen throughout the body. Copper also helps keep bones and nerves healthy.
- Potassium, an important mineral that helps maintain normal fluid and mineral balance, which helps control blood pressure. Potassium also plays a role in making sure nerves and muscles (the heart included!) function properly.
- Beta-glucans, which are antioxidants that help the body resist allergens and strengthen the immune system.

1. Preheat oven to 400°F.

2. Heat oil in a medium ovenproof skillet over medium-high heat. Add mushrooms, stirring occasionally, until just soft, about 5 minutes.

3. Add poblano and cook, stirring occasionally, until mushrooms and poblano are lightly browned, about 5 minutes more. Add kale and scallions, season with salt and pepper, and remove pan from heat.

4. Whisk eggs, cilantro, and cumin in a medium bowl. Season to taste with salt and pepper.

5. Lower heat to medium and pour eggs evenly over mushroom-poblano-kale mixture, using a heatproof spatula to evenly disperse ingredients. Cook until bottom is set, about 2 minutes.

6. Transfer skillet to oven and cook until eggs are just set, about 9 minutes. Remove from oven and let sit 2 minutes.

7. If you don't want to serve the frittata from the pan, you can run a heatproof spatula around the edge of the pan to release frittata. Slide frittata onto a warmed plate and cut into wedges to serve.

KALE, POTATO, AND ONION FRITTATA

MAKES 4 SERVINGS

A frittata is like an open-faced omelet filled with yummy things—in this case, hearty potatoes, savory onions, and delicious kale. You'll need an ovenproof skillet for this one.

1 tablespoon olive oil
1 onion, chopped
1 to 2 cups steamed, cooked, or blanched kale, squeezed dry and chopped
2 cloves garlic, chopped
2 cups boiled diced potatoes
4 whole eggs
  Salt to taste
½ teaspoon paprika

DID YOU KNOW...?

- There are now 200 breeds of chickens.
- Europe has had domesticated hens since 600 BCE.
- An average hen lays 300 to 325 eggs a year. A hen starts laying eggs at 19 weeks of age.
- Chickens came to the New World with Columbus on his second trip in 1493.
- Because eggs are a sign of fertility, French brides break an egg on the threshold of their new home before stepping in.
- In the United States there are approximately 240 million hens, which produce roughly 50 billion eggs each year. That's about one hen for every man, woman, and child in the country.
- White-shelled eggs are produced by hens with white feathers and ear lobes. Brown-shelled eggs are produced by hens with red feathers and red ear lobes.
- There is no difference in nutrition between white and brown eggs.
- To produce one egg, it takes a hen 24–26 hours, and to do so, she requires 5 oz. of food and 10 oz. of water. 30 minutes later she starts all over again.
- Not all eggs have one yolk. Once in awhile, a hen will lay a double-yoked egg. And in rare circumstances, some young hens may produce a yolkless egg.
- Yolk color depends on the diet of the hen. Feed containing yellow corn or alfalfa produces medium yellow yolks, while feed containing wheat or barley produces lighter color yolks.
- As a hen grows older she produces larger eggs.
- A mother hen turns over her egg about fifty times per day (so the yolk won't stick to the sides of the shell).

1. Heat oven to 400°F.

2. In a cast iron or other oven-proof skillet over medium heat, add the olive oil and onion, cooking until onion becomes translucent, about 5 minutes.

3. Add kale and garlic; stir 5 minutes. Add potatoes.

4. In a medium bowl, whisk eggs, egg whites, 2 tablespoons water, salt, and paprika until well mixed.

5. Pour egg mixture over vegetables in skillet. Reduce heat to low and cook for 1 minute just to set the eggs.

POACHED EGGS WITH KALE-CHORIZO HASH

MAKES 2 SERVINGS

This dressy recipe is always a favorite, thanks to flavorful dry-cured chorizo. This is the Spanish type sausage, not the uncured Mexican-style (which is equally delicious!).

2   *tablespoons extra virgin olive oil*
1½ *cups cooked, steamed or blanched kale, squeezed dry and coarsely chopped*
8   *ounces dried Spanish chorizo, halved lengthwise, and then sliced crosswise ¼-inch thick*
2   *eggs*
2   *tablespoons white vinegar*
    Salt and pepper, to taste

1. Add the olive oil to a large skillet over medium heat. Add the chorizo and cook until it has rendered some of its fat, about 3 to 4 minutes.

2. Add the kale, seasoning mixture with salt and pepper and turning kale to coat in chorizo drippings.

3. Make the poached eggs: Pour water into a medium-sized saucepan, filling 3 or 4 inches of water. Bring to a gentle simmer. Once you see tiny bubbles rising from the saucepan, add the vinegar.

4. For the prettiest eggs, crack each egg into its own separate shallow dish. One at a time, gently slide each egg into the gently simmering water, being careful not to break the yolk. (You can use a spoon to coax any migrating egg white back toward the yolk.)

5. As the eggs are cooking (you'll be working quickly, here!), divide the kale-chorizo mixture between two plates.

6. Cook the eggs until the whites have completely set, usually from 2 to 4 minutes.

7. Using a slotted spoon, gently remove, placing each egg on a plate atop the arranged kale-chorizo mixture. Season with salt and pepper as desired. Eat immediately.

EGG NUTRITION

Versatile, inexpensive, and convenient, eggs are one of the nutrient dense foods around. With 75 calories and only 5 grams of fat, eggs are one of the few foods that contain vitamin D, essential for almost all body functions.

A LOOK AT LEEKS

Leeks, the national vegetable of Wales, are also an important part of French, German, Swiss, Austrian, Scottish, Irish, and English cuisines. This is a good thing. Not only do these onion-family favorites lend a rich, satisfying taste to foods, they have proven health benefits, thanks to the following nutrients:

- Soluble and insoluble fiber helps digestive health and cardiovascular health and protects against some cancers.
- Allicin, which laboratory studies show reduces cholesterol while simultaneously having have anti-bacterial, anti-viral, and antifungal benefits.
- B-complex vitamins, such as pyridoxine, folic acid, niacin, riboflavin, and thiamin, all of which assist with healthy nervous system function.
- Vitamin A for healthy eyesight and skin and immune system function.
- Flavonoid anti-oxidants, including carotenes, xanthin, and lutein, which help strengthen the immune system and protect against cancer.
- Vitamin C helps the body develop resistance against infectious agents.
- Vitamin K is essential for cell growth and helps the body maintain healthy blood clotting.
- Vitamin E helps protect the body from invading bacteria and viruses while also strengthening the immune system.
- Small amounts of important minerals such as potassium, iron, calcium, magnesium, manganese, zinc, and selenium.

QUICHE WITH KALE

MAKES 6 TO 8 SERVINGS

This classic-style quiche is a fun way to celebrate morning! It's also a great light supper and travels beautifully to a brunch or lunch potluck. In other words, this quiche is always right!

Your favorite pie or tart dough, fitted into a 9-inch tart pan and blind-baked

1 *cup whole dairy or unsweetened non-dairy milk (or if you have it, ½ cup dairy or non-dairy milk and ½ cup cream or non-dairy cream)*

2 *large eggs plus 1 large egg yolk, room temperature*
  Pinch of freshly grated nutmeg
  Kosher salt and freshly ground pepper to taste

1 *leek, cleaned, chopped and sautéed*

1 *cup cooked, steamed, or blanched kale, squeezed dry and coarsely chopped*

1 *cup grated Gruyère cheese*

1. Heat oven to 375°F.
2. In a medium bowl, stir together the kale and leeks.
3. In another medium bowl, whisk together the milk, eggs, and yolk until combined. Then whisk in the nutmeg and season with salt and pepper.
4. Place the tart pan on a rimmed baking sheet. Sprinkle the bottom of the tart with half of the Gruyère cheese, then with the chopped kale-leek mixture, and then with the remaining half of Gruyère.
5. Carefully pour the custard over the cheese and kale-leek mixture.
6. Bake for about 30 to 35 minutes, until the center is just set.
7. Cool for at least 10 minutes before serving. Serve warm or at room temperature.

IN SEARCH OF A FLUFFY OMELET

As you may already know, an omelet (also spelled omelette) is a dish made from beaten eggs quickly cooked with butter or oil in a frying pan, sometimes folded around a filling such as cheese, vegetables, meat, or some combination of the above. For many cooks, the mark of a good omelet is fluffiness. But how to get this elusive quality? Some cooks beat the eggs to incorporate air bubbles into the eggs. Others add a splash of water, which evaporates (leaving behind bubbles within the omelet's structure). Still others add baking powder to create rise.

QUICHE: THE REAL HISTORY

The word "quiche" is derived from the German word for cake, *kuchen*. Although typically attributed to the French, quiches are actually German in origin. They come from the medieval German kingdom, Lothringen, which was renamed Lorraine when overtaken by the French.

EGGCELLENT!

You've probably seen those omega-enriched eggs at the supermarket. Ever wonder how they got to be so high in these essential fatty acids? It all starts with chicken feed. In other words, whatever the chicken eats a lot of, ends up in her eggs. Thus, many farmers are feeding their chickens flax or chia to increase the amount of both omega-3 and omega-6 fatty acid in eggs.

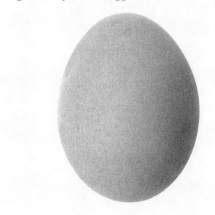

ROASTED RED PEPPER-KALE STRATA

MAKES 6 TO 8 SERVINGS

A strata is a kind of savory bread putting, a terrific way to use stale bread and make eggs stretch further. It's also a terrific make-ahead-and-finish-right-before-serving-brunch kind of dish, one that is so elegant people will think you spent hours on it.

6   *large eggs*
2   *cups half and half or unsweetened non-dairy creamer (such as coconut)*
3   *tablespoons butter or extra virgin olive oil*
1   *cup chopped onion*
½   *cup chopped celery*
1   *cup chopped drained roasted red peppers from jar*
1   *garlic clove, minced*
2   *scallions, chopped*
2   *tablespoons chopped fresh parsley*
1   *teaspoon chopped fresh thyme*
1   *cup cooked, steamed or blanched kale, squeezed dry and coarsely chopped*
8   *cups 1-inch bread cubes from crustless French bread or gluten-free sandwich bread*
1   *teaspoon salt*
¾   *teaspoon ground black pepper*
½   *cup freshly grated Parmesan cheese*

1. Butter 10-inch-diameter cake pan with 2-inch-high sides.
2. Whisk together eggs and half and half in medium bowl to blend.
3. Add olive oil or melt butter in heavy large skillet over medium-high heat. Add onion and celery and sauté until soft, about 5 minutes.
4. Add peppers, garlic, and kale and sauté about 2 minutes.
5. Remove from heat and stir in scallions, parsley, and thyme.
6. Transfer vegetable mixture to large bowl. Add bread cubes and toss to combine.
7. Add whisked egg mixture to vegetable-bread mixture. Season with salt and pepper, mixing well to combine.
8. Transfer mixture to the prepared cake pan. Let stand 30 minutes or cover and refrigerate overnight.
9. When you're ready to cook the strata, preheat oven to 350°F. Sprinkle strata with cheese.
10. Bake until brown and puffed, about 1 hour.
11. Cool on rack 30 minutes. The center will fall, this is normal. Using sharp knife, cut around edge to loosen. Cut into wedges and serve.

SCRAMBLED KALE EGGS

MAKES 2 SERVINGS

This is an easy one, perfect for a fast breakfast on days where you want something healthy. It's a great way to get protein and veggies into your morning. Feel free to increase the kale by a half-cup if you'd like.

1 tablespoon butter or extra virgin olive oil

2 large, fresh eggs

1 cup cooked, steamed, or blanched kale, squeezed dry and chopped shredded kale

Optional: 1 tablespoon milk (dairy or unsweetened non-dairy milk of choice)

Salt and pepper to taste

1. In a small bowl, whisk together eggs, optional milk, and salt and pepper.

2. Add butter or oil to a small skillet over medium heat.

3. Add kale to butter and oil and allow to cook until kale is thoroughly warmed through.

4. Add eggs, stirring and scrambling as they set.

5. Cook until eggs reach your desired state of doneness.

EGG SAFETY AND HANDLING

Want to know how to keep eggs healthy, safe, and delicious to eat? These tips can help:

- An egg can absorb flavors and odors through tiny pores (up to 17,000 of them!) on its surface. Storing eggs in cartons helps keep them fresh.
- As an egg gets older the air space in the egg increases, causing it to float in a bowl of water. Just-laid eggs will always sink in water.
- Eggs are placed in their cartons large end up to keep the air cell in place and the yolk centered.
- Eggs age more in one day at room temperature than in one week in the refrigerator.
- Keep eggs in the main section of the refrigerator at a temperature between 33 and 40°F—eggs accidentally left at room temperature should be discarded after two hours, or one hour in warm weather.
- If kept in a cool refrigerator, eggs can be kept refrigerated in their carton for at least 4 to 5 weeks beyond the pack date.
- A hard-cooked egg will peel more easily if it is a week old before it is cooked.
- To tell if an egg is raw or hard-cooked, spin it! If the egg spins easily, it is hard-cooked, if it wobbles, it is raw.
- A greenish ring around a hard-cooked (boiled) egg yolk can be caused by overcooking or high iron content in the cooking water.
- Eggs are used in recipes to bind, leaven, thicken, emulsify, add protein, and create tenderness.
- Egg whites will beat to a better volume if they're allowed to stand at room temperature for 20 to 30 minutes before beating.

BREAKFAST SANDWICHES

BACON, KALE, AND SWEET POTATO BREAKFAST BURRITOS

MAKES 6 SERVINGS

Breakfast burritos are a fun, delicious, and super-versatile way to get your breakfast greens! Use this recipe as a guide—you can make these without the eggs or meat. You can change up the veggies. You can switch regular potatoes for the sweet potatoes. Try different toppings. Be creative!

3   *slices bacon, chopped*
2½ *cups peeled, cooked sweet potatoes, cubed*
½   *cups red bell pepper, diced*
½   *cups onion, chopped*
1   *cup cooked, steamed, or blanched kale, squeezed dry and coarsely chopped*
4   *eggs*
½   *cups salsa, homemade or purchased*
6   *whole soft flour tortillas*
Optional: ½ cups shredded Jack or mild cheddar cheese
Optional; 1 cup shredded lettuce
Optional: sour cream, cilantro, diced avocado, pepitas, and/or guacamole

1. In a medium bowl, whisk eggs. Set aside

2. Cook bacon in a large skillet over medium heat for about 8 to 10 minutes or until crispy. Remove with a slotted spoon and set aside. Drain bacon fat and reserve.

3. Add one tablespoon reserved bacon fat and cook eggs over medium heat, scrambling until done. Remove eggs and set aside.

4. Add two tablespoons of the reserved bacon fat. Add the bell pepper and onion. Add a couple pinches of salt and pepper over the top and cook, stirring occasionally, for about 5 minutes until the onions begin to soften.

5. Stir in the sweet potatoes and kale. Continue to cook until vegetables are warmed another 5 minutes or so.

6. Remove vegetables to a bowl and get ready salsa, cilantro, tortillas, and optional ingredients.

7. To make breakfast burritos, add about ¼ vegetable filling, a few tablespoons of egg, a few tablespoons of salsa, and desired optional ingredients to the bottom third of a tortilla. Roll or fold tortillas around filling, as desired.

DID YOU KNOW...?

Cilantro is one of the most powerful detoxifying herbs in use today. Health benefits provided by this culinary favorite include:

- Powerful anti-inflammatory capacities that may help symptoms of arthritis
- Protects against bacterial infection from Salmonella in food products
- Has been shown to increase HDL cholesterol (the good kind), and reduces LDL cholesterol (the bad kind)
- Helps relieve stomach gas, prevent flatulence, and works as an overall digestive aid
- Wards off urinary tract infections
- Helps reduce feelings of nausea
- Eases hormonal mood swings associated with menstruation
- Gives relief for diarrhea, especially if caused by microbial or fungal infections
- Helps promote healthy liver function.
- Reduces minor swelling
- Strong general antioxidant properties
- Disinfects and helps detoxify the body
- Stimulates the endocrine glands
- Helps with insulin secretion and lowers blood sugar
- Acts as a natural antiseptic and antifungal agent for skin disorders like fungal infections

EVERYTHING KALE BREAKFAST SANDWICH

MAKES 1 SERVING

This is a yummy, healthy, easy-to-put-together sandwich that is perfect for every day.

1   tablespoon butter or extra virgin olive oil
½   cup cooked, steamed, or blanched kale,
*   squeezed dry and coarsely chopped*
¼   teaspoon paprika
1   egg
1   egg white

2   slices of buttered wheat toast
Optional: 1 to 2 slices cheddar or other cheese

1. Add butter or oil to a medium skillet over medium heat. Add kale and paprika and cook together for 1 or 2 minutes.
2. In a small bowl, whisk together egg and egg white.
3. Pour egg mixture over the kale, allowing eggs to set. Add cheese if using.
4. Flip set eggs if desired.
5. Tuck egg-kale mixture between slices of toast.

KALE TARTINE

MAKES 1 OR 2 SERVINGS

This elegant sandwich is a black tie way to enjoy kale. It's perfect with a mimosa and a side of fresh strawberries.

2   *thick slices of good bread*
2   *tablespoon butter*
½   *cup cooked or steamed kale, squeezed dry and coarsely chopped*
    Salt and pepper to taste
2   *tablespoons chopped chives or mixed herbs of choice*
1   *egg*
    Salt and pepper

1. Toast the bread and scrape on up to one tablespoon of butter.
2. Melt remaining butter in a medium skillet over medium heat.
3. Sautee the kale, herbs, and salt and pepper for a minute, until thoroughly warmed.
4. Add egg and quickly cook until barely scrambled around the kale.
5. Remove from the heat. Season with salt and pepper, pile on the toasted bread, and eat immediately.

WHAT'S A TARTINE?

A tartine is a "dressy" open-faced sandwich with a spread on top. In France, a tartine is usually served with some kind of fancy bread and a complex spread, perhaps topped with a flourish of veggies.

MUFFINS

APPLE AND KALE SPICE MUFFINS

MAKES 12 MUFFINS

This muffin always reminds me of fall. I think it's the apples and the warm cinnamon-nutmeg flavor. This will become a fast favorite. Trust me.

1½ cup whole wheat pastry flour or all-purpose
   flour (you can use a blend)
1   teaspoon each baking soda and baking powder
½   teaspoon salt
1   teaspoon cinnamon
¼   teaspoon nutmeg
1   teaspoon vanilla extract
⅓   cup honey
1   egg
½   cup sour milk or plain unflavored dairy or
   coconut–based yogurt
⅓   cup virgin coconut oil
1½ cup grated apples (you can chop them fine
   in a food processor)
1   cup blanched kale, squeezed dry and finely
   hopped (you can do this in a food processor)
Optional: ½ cup raisins or chopped dried apple
Optional: 1 cup chopped walnuts or pecans

1. Preheat oven to 375°F.
2. Line 12-cup muffin pan with muffin liners.
3. In a large bowl, whisk together flour, baking soda, baking powder, salt, and spices.
4. In another bowl, whisk together honey, egg, yogurt, oil, vanilla, apples, kale, and optional dried fruit and nuts.
5. Add wet ingredients to dry ingredients, stirring just until combined.
6. Fill 12 standard muffin cups ⅔ full. Bake for 18 to 20 minutes, or until muffins are springy to the touch. Allow to cool for 20 minutes before removing.

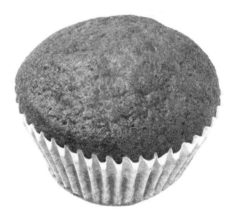

VEGAN "BUTTERMILK"

If you don't use dairy products, you don't have to forgo recipes with buttermilk. Simply make your own vegan buttermilk by adding two tablespoons lemon juice or vinegar to a cup of soy, almond, rice, or other none-dairy milk. Allow milk to sit for 15 minutes and give it a quick whisk before using.

MORNING GLORY KALE MUFFINS

MAKES 12 MUFFINS

Lots of people love those apple and carrot-enriched whole grain muffins called Morning Glory muffins (I know I do!). This is just such a muffin, with the addition of (shhh!!!) kale. You'll love it, as will everyone else. Though you may want to keep the kale on the low-down, if you know what I mean.

¼   cup orange juice

¼   cup virgin coconut oil

½   cup agave syrup

1   egg

½   cup milk or unsweetened non-dairy milk (I like almond milk in this recipe)

1   teaspoon vanilla or almond extract

½   cup shredded carrots

½   cup kale, cooked, steamed, or blanched 'til tender then pureed with 2 tablespoons almond milk in food processor

1½   cup whole wheat pastry flour

½   teaspoon nutmeg or cinnamon

1   teaspoon baking soda

1   teaspoon baking powder

Optional: ½ cup chopped walnuts or other nuts

Optional: ½ cup raisins or dried cranberries or dried blueberries or fresh blueberries

1. Preheat oven to 375°F.

2. Prepare 12 standard muffin tins by fitting with cupcake liners.

3. In a food processor, puree kale with two tablespoons or so of the milk.

4. In a large bowl, sift together flour, nutmeg, baking soda, baking powder, and salt.

5. In the bowl of the food processor, add juice, coconut oil, syrup, egg, milk, and vanilla extract, pulsing ingredients until smooth.

6. Add liquid ingredients to dry ingredients, mixing only until combined.

7. Fold carrots and any optional ingredients to batter, being careful not to overmix.

8. Fill prepared muffin cups ⅔ full with batter. Bake for 17 to 22 minutes, or until muffins are springy to the touch. Allow finished muffins to cool 20 minutes or so before removing.

SAVORY CARROT AND KALE MUFFINS (grain-free/gluten-free)

MAKES 12 MUFFINS

I like this recipe because it's not sweet. Sometimes I think I am one of the only people in North America who doesn't like to have sweet foods for breakfast! It's also great tasting, healthy, and doesn't contain gluten, a real plus for my gluten-free sons.

2   cups blanched almond flour
½   cup coconut flour
1¼ teaspoons baking powder
1   teaspoon baking soda
1   teaspoon salt
1   or 2 teaspoons dried thyme
1   or 2 teaspoons dried basil
1   cup carrot, finely grated
1   cup blanched kale, squeezed dry and finely chopped
4   eggs
¼   cup honey
1   cup virgin coconut oil
½   cup dairy or non-dairy yogurt (I like plain coconut yogurt in this recipe)

1. Preheat oven to 350°F.
2. Line two 12-cup muffin pans with muffin liners.
3. In a large bowl, whisk together almond and coconut flours, baking powder, baking soda and salt, thyme, and basil.
4. Add carrots and kale to dry ingredients and mix together until everything is thoroughly combined.
5. In a food processor or high-speed blender (such as a VitaMix), add eggs and honey. Process for 20 seconds.
6. Add coconut oil and yogurt to the food processor or blender and process an additional 20 seconds until all ingredients are combined and the mixture is smooth.
7. Pour wet ingredients into dry ingredients, mixing until thoroughly combined.
8. Fill muffin cups ⅔ full and bake for 18 to 20 minutes, or until muffins are springy to the touch. Cool for 20 minutes before removing muffins from pan.

BAKING WITHOUT GLUTEN

Gluten, the protein in wheat, gives baked goods structure and a soft, springy texture. If you've been told you have to give up gluten, you have options, one of them being chia. Just keep in mind that baked goods made without wheat may have either a heavier moisture, or a drier texture, depending upon the non-gluten flour you bake with.

CINNAMON'S SWEET BENEFITS

- Cinnamon has a lot of fans, most recently among researchers who have been diligently studying its health-supportive properties. Some of the most impressive of these, include: ½ teaspoon of cinnamon per day can lower your bad cholesterol (LDL).
- Cinnamon may help treat Type 2 Diabetes by lowering blood sugar levels and increasing the amount of insulin production in the body.
- Cinnamon has an anti-clotting effect on the blood.
- Cinnamon has antifungal properties, and it's been said that Candida cannot live in the presence of cinnamon. Candida, known more formally as Candida albicans, is a yeast organism found in low levels in healthy bodies. In some individuals, it can "over-grow," leading to thrush, vaginitis, digestive upset or severe rectal itching.
- Cinnamon can reduce the proliferation of leukemia and lymphoma cancer cells.
- When added to food, cinnamon inhibits bacterial growth and food spoilage, making it a natural food preservative.
- Studies have found that the act of smelling cinnamon boosts cognitive function and memory.
- Cinnamon has been found to be an effective natural remedy for eliminating headaches and migraine relief.

SUMMER SQUASH-KALE MUFFINS

MAKES 12 MUFFINS

This yummy recipe is reminiscent of zucchini bread, that summertime staple in gardening homes. It's an easy, fun, portable breakfast on the go and makes a delicious mid-morning snack.

1½ cups grated fresh zucchini or yellow squash
1 cup cooked or steamed kale, coarsely chopped
2 eggs
1 cup sugar
1 teaspoon vanilla
¼ cup virgin coconut oil
¼ cup applesauce, pearsauce or pumpkin puree
2 teaspoons baking soda
1 pinch salt
3 cups whole wheat pastry or all-purpose flour (you can use a mix)
1 to 2 teaspoons cinnamon (or a mixture of cinnamon, ginger, nutmeg, cloves, and/or allspice)
Optional: 1 cup chopped walnuts, pecans, or other nuts

1. Preheat oven to 350°F.
2. Prepare a 12-cup standard muffin tin or 24-cup mini muffin tin with cupcake liners.
3. In a large bowl, whisk eggs.
4. Add sugar, vanilla, oil, and applesauce,

mixing until combined and beat until sugar is dissolved and mixture is light in color.

5. Fold in zucchini and kale, thoroughly combining.

6. In a large bowl, whisk together all remaining ingredients but nuts.

7. Add dry ingredients to wet ingredients, mixing just until combined. Gently fold in optional nuts, being careful not to overmix.

8. Fill muffin cups ⅔ full with batter and bake for 15 to 20 minutes for mini muffins, 25 to 30 minutes for standard muffins, or until muffins are springy to the touch. Let cool for 20 minutes before removing from pan.

EASY LEMON ZEST

I love the bright zing that fresh lemon zest brings food. But zesting lemons is not fun—unless you have a plane grater. These hand-held, wand-like graters make fast work of lemon zest. Try one and you'll wonder how you survived without one.

SUPER AWESOME HEALTH MUFFINS

MAKE 9 LARGE MUFFINS

These gorgeous muffins have all kinds of healthy things in them, including blueberries! My hubby loves one of these with his afternoon coffee.

1   cup whole wheat pastry flour or all-purpose flour
¾   cup golden flaxseed meal
½   cup brown sugar
1   tablespoon baking powder
1   teaspoon cinnamon or lemon zest
½   teaspoon salt
1   cup plain yogurt (can use coconut or other non-dairy yogurt)
2   tablespoons virgin coconut oil
1   egg, lightly beaten
1   cup cooked, steamed, or blanched kale, squeezed dry and finely chopped
1   cup fresh or frozen blueberries

1. Preheat oven to 375°F.

2. Prepare 9 muffin cups by lining muffin tin with cupcake liners

3. In a medium bowl, whisk together four, flaxseed meal, brown sugar, baking powder, and cinnamon.

4. In another bowl, whisk together the yogurt, coconut oil, and egg.

5. Pour the wet ingredients into the dry ingredients, stirring only to combine.

6. Add blueberries and kale, gently folding them into the batter. Be careful not to overmix.

7. Fill muffin cups ⅔ full and bake for 20 to 25 minutes or until muffins are springy to the touch. Allow them to cool for 20 minutes before removing them.

VEGAN BANANA-KALE MUFFINS

MAKES 6 MUFFINS

This easy eggless recipe is super versatile. Add chocolate chips, chopped nuts, even diced dried fruit. If you don't have whole wheat pastry flour, use regular unbleached all-purpose flour.

3   *medium ripe bananas*
4   *raw kale leaves, deribbed*
¼   *cup virgin coconut oil*
1   *cup sugar*
2   *cups whole wheat pastry flour*
½   *teaspoon cinnamon*
½   *teaspoons sea salt*
1   *teaspoon baking soda*

1. Fit a 6-cup standard muffin tin or 12-cup mini-muffin tin with cupcake liners.
2. Preheat oven to 350°F.
3. In the bowl of a food processor or high-speed blender, place the bananas and kale leaves. Pulse a few times until kale has been pulverized.
4. Add the oil and sugar and blend until smooth.
5. In large bowl, whisk together the whole wheat pastry flour, cinnamon, salt, and baking soda.
6. Pour the wet ingredients into the dry ingredients and mix just to combine, being careful not to overmix the batter.
7. Fill prepared muffin cups ⅔ full and bake for 15 minutes or until they are springy to the touch and a toothpick comes out clean.

ABOUT THE WORD "MUFFIN"

The name "muffin" is thought to come from the French word *moufflet*, meaning soft bread.

CEREAL

IRISH OATS

MAKES 2 SERVINGS

This recipe makes one bowl of very (very) green porridge. My kids will happily eat this on St. Paddy's Day, but avoid it on other, less Irish days of the year. Go figure.

½   cups water
     Dash of salt
1   cup steel cut oats
1   cup blanched kale
½   cup almond milk
¼   cup unsweetened applesauce
¼   cup unsweetened coconut flakes
3   tablespoons maple syrup
Optional: Chopped walnuts

1. In a medium pot, bring water to boil. Add a dash of salt.
2. Add oats to the boiling water. Lower heat and cook for 20 to 30 minutes.
3. While the oats are cooking, add kale, almond milk, applesauce, coconut, and maple syrup to a high-speed blender, such as a Vita-Mix. Process until completely liquefied.
4. Bring the heat up to medium-high on the oats. Pour in the green mixture and add the coconut flakes. Continue cooking until thick.
5. To serve, spoon into a bowl and sprinkle chopped walnuts on top.

YAY, OATMEAL

Oatmeal comes from the grain of the oat plant. After harvesting, oats are minimally processed—the manufacturer removes the hull of the oat grain and grinds the grain into coarse flakes. A one-cup serving of oatmeal contains 311 calories and the following percentages of the recommended daily value of these nutrients:

- 32% of dietary fiber
- 26% of protein
- 39% of thiamin
- 38% of phosphorus

- 30% of magnesium
- 19% of iron
- 14% of copper

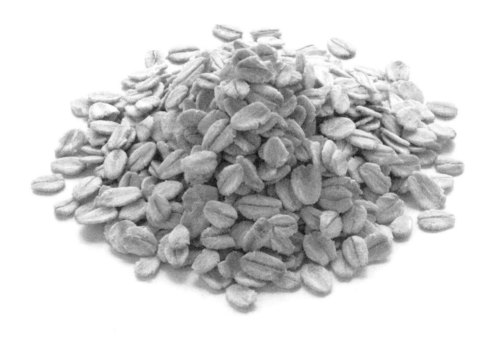

HOTCAKES

DINER-STYLE KALE PANCAKES

MAKES ABOUT 8 MEDIUM-SIZED PANCAKES

This is a natural for St. Paddy's Day, is the perfect accompaniment to Green Eggs and Ham, and is fun for any kid who likes green. Plus, they taste good!

2   *cups of whole wheat pastry flour or gluten-free all-purpose flour blend*

1   *tablespoon of ground chia*

1   *teaspoon of salt*

2   *tablespoons of sugar*

1¾ *tablespoons of baking powder*

Optional: 1 teaspoon cinnamon or a mix of cinnamon, ginger, nutmeg, cloves, and allspice

4   *tablespoons virgin coconut oil*

8   *tablespoons of applesauce or pumpkin puree*

2   *eggs*

TENDER PANCAKES EVERY TIME

For tender pancakes, go easy on the blending. Whisk together the dry ingredients and the wet ingredients separately, then combine them. Mixing only until just barely incorporated. Stop immediately once that happens!

1½ *cup of dairy or nondairy milk*

½   *cup cooked, steamed or blanched kale, pureed*

½   *teaspoon vanilla*

1. In a large bowl, whisk together flour, chia, salt, sugar, baking powder, and optional spices.
2. In a separate bowl, whisk together oil, applesauce, eggs, milk, kale puree, and vanilla.
3. Add the liquid ingredients to the flour mixture, stirring only until combined and being careful not to overmix.
4. Cook on a nonstick griddle placed over medium-high heat.

PANCAKE FUN

- Some countries celebrate Mardi Gras (aka Shrove Tuesday) as Pancake Day. What better excuse to enjoy some buttery, super sweet, rich food before Lent?
- Pancakes begin appearing in written recipes and cookbooks in the very early 1400s.
- Once upon a time there was no such thing as pancake mix. Then, in 1889, the world's first ready-made mix was sold commercially. Its name? Aunt Jemima Pancake Flour, invented in St. Joseph, Missouri.
- Pancake breakfasts are a favorite fundraising activity. The world's largest of these happened in 1999 in Springfield, Massachusetts, with more than 71,233 servings of pancakes being served to over 40,000 people. If you stacked up all those pancakes, they'd be more than 2 miles high!

KALE WAFFLES

MAKES ABOUT 8 MEDIUM WAFFLES

Most of us have fond memories of our mothers or grandmothers making us waffles—or even ordering waffles in a diner or pancake house. Nowadays, however, we're so busy that most of us rely on prepackaged frozen waffles. I'm here to tell you that if you have a waffle iron, waffles are fast and easy to make. Plus, you can freeze a few for another day, creating your own stash of frozen breakfast treats!

1¾ cup almond, hemp or coconut milk
3   eggs
1   cup chopped raw kale leaves
¼   cup virgin coconut oil
1   teaspoon vanilla extract
1   teaspoon salt
1   teaspoon cinnamon
2   cups whole wheat pastry flour or gluten-free all-purpose flour blend
2   teaspoons baking powder

1. Plug in your waffle iron and set it to medium heat.
2. Place milk, kale, oil, vanilla, and salt in a high-speed blender, such as a VitaMix. Blend until liquefied.
3. Add cinnamon, flour, and baking powder to the VitaMix and pulse just until blended (being careful to not overmix).
4. To prevent deflated waffles, let batter sit 5 to 10 minutes before pouring in waffle iron.
5. Use waffle batter to make waffles per your waffle maker's instructions.

WAFFLE STACK

Looking for something different for breakfast? Take a frozen or homemade waffle, top it with a serving of scrambled egg, a thin red onion slice, ¼ cup of kale, an optional flourish of grated cheese, and pop into a toaster oven set on broil. Remove when cheese has melted. Serve as-is or with a splash of hot sauce or tablespoon of salsa. Yum!

SAVORY WAFFLES

MAKES ABOUT 4 MEDIUM WAFFLES

Sometimes you want something hearty and savory for breakfast. For those times, try these delicious waffles.

¾   cup whole wheat pastry flour or gluten-free all-purpose flour blend
¼   cup cornmeal
¼   teaspoon salt
1½   baking powder
¾   cup dairy or unsweetened nondairy milk
1   egg
½   cup cheddar cheese, shredded
½   cup cooked kale, squeezed dry and coarsely chopped
4   slices ham or other meat, chopped
     Ketchup, salsa, or other condiments for serving

1. Plug in your waffle iron and set it to medium heat.

2. In a large bowl, whisk together flour, cornmeal, salt, and baking powder.

3. In a separate bowl, whisk milk and egg until incorporated.

4. Stir liquid ingredients into dry ingredients, mixing only until combined.

5. Gently fold in meat, cheese, and kale, being careful not to over mix.

6. Use waffle batter to make waffles per your waffle maker's instruction.

A LOOK BACK

Waffles have a long and glorious history. The ancient Greeks used to cook a waffle-like something called *oblelios*, a type of flat cake cooked between two metal plates. By the Middle Ages, the Europeans were making *oblelios*, sometimes in their original flat form and sometimes rolled into cones. It wasn't until the 13th century, however, that decorated waffle plates appeared, changing the look of waffles as we know them!

LYCO-WHAT?

If you're a tomato lover, you may know about lycopene, an antioxidant in the carotenoid family that is present in tomatoes. This red, fat-soluble pigment helps neutralize harmful free radicals, which are implicated in cancer, heart disease, macular degeneration, and other age-related illnesses. It also helps protect the body against cancer.

Lycopene is especially high in cooked tomato products. Why? Cooking processed tomatoes breaks down cell walls, releasing and concentrating carotenoids. Ketchup, canned tomato soup, tomato juice, pasta sauce, and pizza sauce, are the richest sources of lycopene.

MORNING POTATOES

CHORIZO KALE HASH BROWNS

MAKES 4 TO 6 SERVINGS

I love potatoes, especially during the cold weather months when a body craves something filling. That said, I don't eat a lot of them—I'm one of those sensitive types whose blood sugar goes crazy after just one serving of the starchy tubers. However, I've found that by combining potatoes with protein and greens, sensitive people like me are much better able to enjoy the comforting veggie.

1   *medium onion, finely chopped*
1   *or 2 garlic cloves, minced*
2   *tablespoons extra-virgin olive oil, divided*
2   *pounds russet (baking) potatoes (about 3), peeled*
2   *ounces Spanish chorizo (cured spiced pork sausage), finely chopped (about ½ cup)*
½   *cup cooked or steamed kale, squeezed dry and finely chopped*
¼   *cup chopped flat-leaf parsley*
    Dash of paprika
½   *teaspoon salt*
    Dash black pepper
1   *tablespoon unsalted butter*

1. Add 1 tablespoon oil to a nonstick skillet and, over medium heat, sauté onion, and garlic until softened, about 3 to 5 minutes.

2. Using a box grater or the grating attachment of a food processor, coarsely grate potatoes. Squeeze out any excess water.

3. In a large bowl, mix together cooked onion mixture, grated potatoes, chorizo, kale, parsley, paprika, salt, and pepper until thoroughly combined.

4. Wipe out the skillet and heat butter and remaining tablespoon of oil over medium heat until butter is melted.

5. Add mixture, spreading it evenly in skillet and pressing gently to flatten. Cook over medium heat until crisp and golden, 8 to 10 minutes.

6. To turn the hash brown, invert a large plate over skillet. Holding plate and skillet tightly together, invert hash browns onto plate. Slide the hash browns back into skillet and press gently to flatten. Cook until golden and cooked through, 8 to 10 minutes more. Cut into wedges and serve.

HASH WHAT POTATOES?

While some people say hash browns originated from the Swiss potato dish rösti, hash brown potatoes are as American as apple pie, showing up in the American food lexicon in 1888, when food author Maria Parloa mentions "hashed browned potatoes." The name was gradually shortened to "hash brown potatoes." By the late 1960s, people were merely saying "hash browns."

OVEN HASH KALE CAKES

MAKES 4 SERVINGS

This oven recipe is a glorified potato pancake—as yummy and satisfying as any you've ever had, with the healthy addition of kale.

> *Butter for greasing pan*
> 1½ cups paper-thin onion slices, preferably from a sweet onion such as Vidalia
> 1 pound Yukon Gold potatoes, peeled
> ¼ cup cooked or steamed kale, squeezed dry and chopped finely
> 1 teaspoon salt, divided
> 2 tablespoons unsalted butter, melted

1. Preheat oven to 425°F.

2. Grease a large rimmed nonstick baking sheet with butter.

3. Using a box grater or the grating attachment of a food processor, coarsely grate potatoes.

4. Toss potatoes with ½ teaspoon salt in medium bowl. Let stand 5 minutes. Using hands, squeeze out excess liquid from potatoes.

5. Place onion in large bowl. Add potatoes, kale, ½ teaspoon salt, and melted butter. Toss to coat.

6. Divide mixture into 4 mounds on prepared baking sheet, allowing space between mounds.

7. Roast 15 minutes, then turn mounds over with spatula, pressing down to flatten to 4-inch-diameter rounds (cakes will still be soft).

8. Reduce oven temperature to 350°F and bake until cakes are golden and crisp around edges, about 45 minutes longer.

POTATOES YOUR WAY

- Home fries are a basic potato preparation featured cubed potatoes cooked in oil or fat.
- Rösti is a Swiss shredded potato dish, traditionally eaten as a "farmer's breakfast."
- Potato pancakes feature shredded potato and egg, cooked in the shape of a griddle cake.
- Corned beef hash contains cubed or shredded potatoes fried with onions and corned beef.
- Potatoes O'Brien are hash browns cooked with green bell peppers.
- Tater Tots is a trademark name for a form of small shredded potato puffs.
- Potato waffles are waffle-shaped frozen potato cakes sold in the UK and Ireland.
- Hash is a dish made of fried potato and bits of leftover meat and veggies.
- Bubble and squeak potato contains potatoes, fried together with leftovers.
- Rappie pie is a French-North American casserole made with shredded potatoes.
- Boxty is a popular Irish potato dish.
- Croquettes are small fried items bound with mashed potatoes.
- Aloo tikki is a North Indian potato snack.

POTATO AND KALE GALETTE

MAKES 8 SERVINGS

I don't have superlatives enough for this elegant dish. All I can say is you must try it. Very soon. In order to slice the potatoes super-thin, you'll need a mandoline, or a food processor fitted with a slicing blade. You'll also need a super heavy large skillet, such as a cast iron pan, to use as a weight.

4 *garlic cloves, finely chopped*
2 *cups cooked or steamed kale, squeezed dry*
   and coarsely chopped.
1 *stick (½ cup) butter, 6 tablespoons melted*
   and cooled
2 *pounds russet (baking) potatoes (4 medium),*
   peeled
¾ *teaspoon salt*
¾ *teaspoon black pepper*
   Paprika

1. Heat 2 tablespoons of the unmelted butter in a large nonstick skillet over medium-high heat. Add garlic and cook, stirring occasionally, until golden, about one minute.

2. To the skillet add kale, ¼ teaspoon salt, and ¼ teaspoon pepper. Sauté until kale is warmed through, about 2 to 4 minutes.

3. Transfer kale mixture to a bowl and wipe out skillet.

4. Using a mandoline or a food processor outfitted with a slicing blade, slice potatoes crosswise no more than ¹⁄₁₆ of an inch thick.

5. Working quickly to prevent potatoes from discoloring, generously brush bottom of skillet with some of melted butter and cover with ⅓ of the potato slices, overlapping slightly. Dab potatoes with some of melted butter.

6. Spread half of kale over potatoes and sprinkle with ⅛ teaspoon salt and ⅛ teaspoon pepper.

BLACK PEPPER: NOTHING TO SNEEZE AT

Black pepper has a reputation as a sneeze-maker, thanks to the way small bits of the spice can enter and irritate the nasal cavity. Fortunately, this is more annoying than harmful, for black pepper has so many health benefits, you'll want to use it often:

- A two-teaspoon dose of black pepper contains 12% of your daily requirement of manganese, 8.6% of vitamin K, 6.7% of iron, 4.4.% of fiber, and 2.5% of copper.
- Black pepper is a carminative, a substance that helps prevent the formation of intestinal gas.
- Black pepper has diaphoretic properties, meaning it promotes sweating.
- It also is a diuretic, helping the body flush excess water through urination.
- It has powerful antibacterial effects, making it an important ingredient to help stay healthy.

7. Cover with half of remaining potato slices and dab with butter, then top with remaining kale. Sprinkle with ⅛ teaspoon salt and ⅛ teaspoon pepper. Top with remaining potatoes and sprinkle with remaining ¼ teaspoon salt and ¼ teaspoon pepper. Finish, if desired, with a dusting of paprika.

8. Brush a sheet of foil with melted butter, then brush galette with any remaining butter and place foil, buttered side down, on top. Place a 10-inch heavy skillet on top of foil to weight galette.

9. Cook galette over moderate heat until underside is golden brown, about 12 to 15 minutes. Remove top skillet and foil. Wearing oven mitts, carefully slide galette onto a baking sheet and invert skillet over it. Holding them together, invert galette, browned side up, back into skillet. Cook, uncovered, over moderate heat until underside is golden brown and potatoes are tender, 12 to 15 minutes. Slide onto a serving plate.

10. If you'd like, you can make the galette 4 or 5 hours ahead. Cool the cooked galette. Once it's cool, you can place it on a baking sheet covered with foil, allowing it to sit out at room temperature. To reheat, remove foil, then warm the galette in a 400°F oven until heated through and crisp, about 20 minutes.

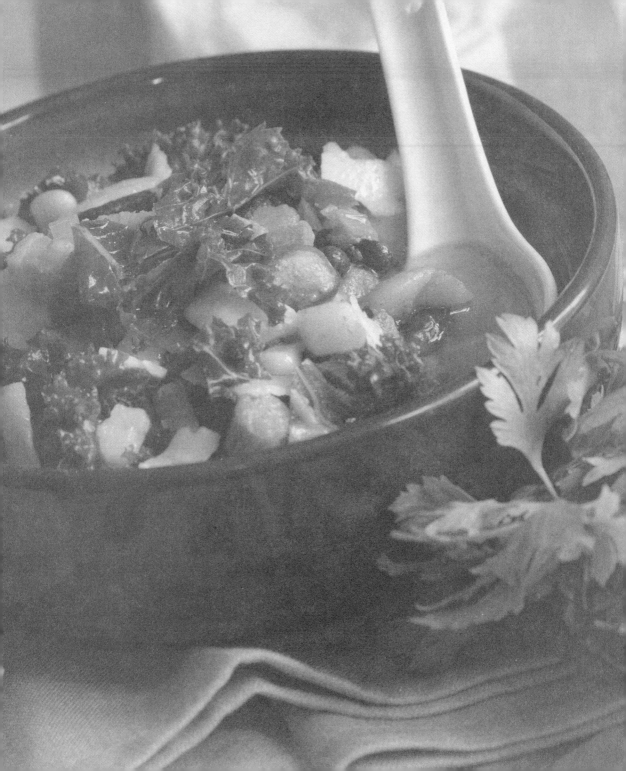

CHAPTER 5

KALE FOR LUNCH

You know that old saying about breakfast being the most important meal of the day? For me, the most important meal of the day is lunch. Without a doubt. Midday is when your body is busiest, needing the most calories to fuel it through a marathon of mental and physical (even emotional) activities.

One wrong turn, and you can choose a meal that will make you sluggish, or put you on a cycle of cravings, or upset your tummy, or leave you spacey, or make you irritable, or create some other kind of outcome that will hamper your ability to be productive and creative.

Done right, lunch can energize you and leave you feeling satisfied, happy, intellectually sharp, happy, and powerful. Kale can help with that. Really. Sometimes when I am feeling sluggish and mentally slow, I add a green juice made with kale to my lunch menu. Or, I'll juice a soup or salad featuring kale. Afterward, I feel focused and clear-headed, ready to tackle anything that makes its way across my desk.

Try it for yourself. I dare you: Today (or tomorrow), have kale for lunch and see how great you feel afterward!

SOUPS, STEWS, AND CHILIS

BARLEY-KALE STEW
MAKES 6 SERVINGS

This hearty, meatless stew is satisfying as well as deeply healing thanks to the bountiful antioxidants found in barley, kale, leeks, tomatoes, garlic, and tomato—all ingredients in this yummy recipe.

1   *tablespoon olive oil, divided*
2   *small leeks, chopped (white and pale green parts only)*
1½   *cups thinly sliced button or cremini mushrooms (you can use a mix)*
2   *garlic cloves, minced*
2¼   *teaspoons minced fresh rosemary*
1   *(14.5-ounce) can diced tomatoes in juice*
1   *cup pearl barley*
4   *cups (or more) chicken or vegetable broth*
1   *bunch kale, deribbed and coarsely chopped*

1. Heat oil in heavy large pot over medium heat. Add leeks; sprinkle with salt and pepper and sauté until leeks begin to soften, stirring often, about 5 minutes.

2. Add mushrooms, garlic, and rosemary; increase heat to medium-high and sauté until mushrooms soften and begin to brown, stirring often, about 7 minutes.

3. Add tomatoes with their juice; stir 1 minute.

4. Add barley and 4 cups broth. Bring to boil.

5. Reduce heat to low, cover, and simmer until barley is almost tender, about 20 to 30 minutes.

6. Add kale. Cover and simmer until kale and barley are tender, about 15 minutes. Note: if you desire a more liquid consistency, add ¼ cup or more broth as desired.

GETTING TO KNOW BARLEY

Barley is a nourishing cereal grain rich in fiber, protein, and B-complex vitamins. Cultivated since ancient times, it is enjoyed in many different forms:

- **Hulled barley:** Chewy and dense, hulled barley is a whole grain that has only its outermost husk removed.
- **Scotch barley:** Also called pot barley, grains are polished to remove the outer hull. Not as dense, chewy, or nutritious as hulled barley, Scotch barley is still a high-nutrient food. Its name comes from Scotland, where it was and is a popular soup pot ingredient.
- **Pearl barley:** By polishing, or "pearling" grains of barley, the outermost hull, the grain's brain layer and even part of its inner endosperm layer, are all removed. Quicker cooking and lighter in texture than hulled barley, pearl barley is markedly lower in nutrients.
- **Barley flakes:** Think rolled oats—only with barley. Eaten as a hot cereal or added to baked goods.
- **Barley grits:** Hulled, Scotch, or even pearl barley can be toasted and cracked, creating what is known as barley grits. These can be cooked and eaten as a breakfast cereal or a side dish with meats and veggies.

CANNELINI-BUTTERNUT-KALE STEW

MAKES 6 SERVINGS

For me, butternut squash means autumn. I love roasted the squash and pureeing it into smoothies, sauces, and soups, or cutting into chunks and tossing with oil and herbs before roasting. In this warming recipe, this well-loved squash is joined by kale and white beans.

¼ cup olive oil

3 large onions, chopped

6 garlic cloves, minced

1 2- to 3-pound butternut squash, peeled, seeded, cut into 1½-inch cubes

3 red or orange bell peppers, seeded, cut into 1½-inch pieces

1½ cups chicken broth

1½ large bunches kale, deribbed and coarsely chopped

½ tablespoon dried rubbed sage

¼ teaspoon red pepper flakes

5 (15-ounce) cans cannellini (white kidney beans), rinsed, drained

Optional: Grated parmesan cheese, chopped parsley

1. Heat oil in heavy large Dutch oven over medium-high heat. Add onions and garlic; sauté until tender, about 10 minutes.

2. Add squash; sauté.

3. Add bell peppers and stir to coat with onion mixture. Add broth. Cover and simmer until squash is just tender, about 10 minutes.

4. Mix kale, sage, and red pepper flakes into stew. Cover and cook until kale wilts, stirring occasionally, about 8 minutes.

5. Add beans and stir until heated through. Season to taste with salt and pepper.

6. Serve with optional toppings.

HEALING WITH OLIVES

For years health advocates have been talking about the benefits olive oil—how it lowers cholesterol, helps with blood pressure, and even strengthens the immune system. Whole olives are just as healing. In fact, herbalists have long used preparations from olives and olive leaves to treat inflammatory conditions and allergies.

How do they work? Olive extracts function as antihistamines at a cellular level. Histamines are molecules that create inflammation. Thus, olives—your favorite cured olives!—are a wonderful addition to anyone's diet, especially those of you who suffer from environmental, food, or contact allergies.

CANNELLINI BEANS

Popular in Tuscany, cannellini beans are large white beans, with a firm texture and skin and a nut-like flavor. I love their versatility—they hold their shape well, making them great for salads. They are delicious in soup. And they are outstanding pureed with roasted garlic as a sandwich spread or dip. Want to get to know the cannellini better? Here's some fun facts about the bean:

- Cannellini are related to kidney beans, great northern, navy, and green beans, among others.
- Like other beans, cannellinies are low in fat and high in protein, fiber, minerals, and B vitamins.
- The Tuscans so love cannellini beans that the people are referred to as "bean eaters," or "mangiafagioli" in Italian.
- Some people call cannellini beans "white kidney beans."
- Cannellinies are a traditional ingredient in minestrone.
- One cup of the beans contain 20 grams of protein, 12 grams of fiber, 20 percent of an adult's daily requirement of iron and 8 percent of an adult's daily requirement of calcium.

KALE AND CANNELLINI SOUP

MAKES 6 SERVINGS

If you're a recipe collector—and there are a lot of us in the world—I know you've come across several recipes that feature the classic combo of kale and cannellini beans. It's a delicious, nutritious, hearty combination that is as beautiful to look at as it is wonderful to eat. Here, kale and cannellini find their way into the same soup pot with pancetta, chestnut, and parmesan!

½ *pound dried cannellini beans (about 1¼ cups), picked over and rinsed*
¼ *pound thinly sliced pancetta, chopped*
1 *large onion, chopped*
3 *garlic cloves, minced*
3 *tablespoons extra-virgin olive oil*
1 *(14-ounce) can diced tomatoes, juice reserved*
3½ *cups chicken broth*
2 *cups water*
1 *piece Parmigiano-Reggiano rind (roughly 3- by 3-inch)*
   Salt and pepper to taste
1½ *cups bottled peeled cooked whole chestnuts (8 ounces), halved*
½ *pound kale (preferably Lacinto), deribbed and roughly chopped*
2 *teaspoons chopped fresh thyme*
Optional garnish: Parmigiano-Reggiano shavings, black pepper

1. Soak beans in cold water to cover by 2 inches in a bowl at room temperature at least 8 hours. Drain well in a colander.

2. In a large, heavy pot over moderate heat, sauté pancetta, onion, and garlic in olive oil. Stir occasionally, cooking until browned, about 8 minutes.

3. Add tomatoes with juice, beans, broth, water, cheese rind, salt, and pepper and simmer, uncovered, until beans are tender, 45 minutes to 1 hour. Remove cheese rind.

4. Stir in chestnuts.

5. Transfer 2½ cups soup to a blender and purée until smooth. Return to the pot.

6. Stir in kale and simmer, uncovered, stirring occasionally, until leaves are tender, 10 to 15 minutes.

7. Stir in thyme.

HEALTH BENEFITS OF CHESTNUT

Chestnuts aren't like all those other nuts. They're starchier. Higher in vitamins. (In fact, their nutrition composition is very similar to sweet potatoes!) And they are loaded with minerals and phytonutrients. Want to know more? Here you go:

- Chestnuts are a good source of dietary fiber, providing 21% of daily recommended value per 100-gram serving. As you may know, fiber helps with digestion and lowers blood cholesterol levels by limiting excess cholesterol absorption in the intestines.

- Chestnuts are rich in vitamin C, with 72% of daily recommended value per 100-gram serving. Vitamin C strengthens the immune system and, as an antioxidant, it offers protection from harmful free radicals.

- Unlike other nuts and seeds, chestnuts are rich in folic acid. A 100-gram serving provides 15.5% of the daily recommended value. Folic acid is required for the formation of red blood cells and DNA synthesis, making it an essential during pregnancy.

- Chestnuts are rich source of mono-unsaturated fatty like oleic acid and palmitoleic acids. Studies suggest that monounsaturated fats in the diet help lower LDL (bad cholesterol) and increase HDL (good cholesterol) levels within the blood.

- Further, they are also rich in many important B-complex groups of vitamins, helpful for healthy nervous system function. A 100-gram serving of chestnuts provide 11% of niacin, 29% of pyridoxine (vitamin B-6), 100% of thiamin, and 12% of riboflavin.

- The nut is also an excellent source of minerals such as iron, calcium, magnesium, manganese, phosphorus, potassium, and zinc.

GARBANZO KALE SOUP

MAKES 6 TO 8 SERVINGS

This warming soup features one of my favorite flavor duos: chickpea and kale. One is mellow and nutty-tasting, while the other is a bit brassy and astringent. Both have a meaty bite and are outrageously healthy!

2   tablespoons extra-virgin olive oil
1   medium onion, chopped
2   garlic cloves, minced
    Salt and pepper to taste
1   bay leaf
2   medium red-skinned (boiling) potatoes, peeled and cut into ½-inch cubes
¾   pound kale, deribbed, leaves finely chopped
5½ cups chicken broth
1   (14-ounce) can chickpeas, rinsed and drained
¼   pound Spanish chorizo (cured spiced pork sausage), casing removed and sausage cut into ¼-inch dice (about 1 cup)

1. In a large, heavy pot over medium heat, sauté onion, garlic, salt, and pepper in oil, stirring frequently, until onion and garlic are softened and beginning to brown, about 5 to 7 minutes.

2. Add bay leaf, potato, kale, broth, and water and cook, partially covered, until potatoes are tender, 15 to 20 minutes.

3. Reduce heat to low, then add chickpeas and chorizo and gently simmer, uncovered, for about 3 to 5 minutes.

4. Remove bay leaf and season with salt and pepper.

> ### GO GO GARBANZOS!
>
> Garbanzos, also known as chickpeas, contain about 12.5 grams of fiber per cup. That's 50% of the daily recommended value. This explains why participants in a recent study reported more satisfaction with their diet when garbanzo beans were included, consuming fewer processed food snacks and less food overall. Bring on the hummus!

LENTIL AND VEGETABLE STEW WITH KALE

MAKES 8 SERVINGS

We use a lot of lentils in my house. They are inexpensive (important when feeding three boys, a couple who need costly special food), fast to cook, mild-tasting and incredibly versatile. Oh, and they are also nutritional, filled with protein and fiber. This soup is simple way to get more of this little legume into your daily diet.

2   tablespoons olive oil
1   large onion, chopped
2   large carrots, peeled and cut into large dice
1   to 2 large celery stalks, chopped
    Salt and pepper to taste
1   medium rutabaga, peeled and cut into large dice
1   to 2 garlic cloves, minced

1   *pound brown lentils, rinsed*
1   *tablespoon herbes de Provence*
8   *cups (or more) chicken or vegetable broth*
1   *large bunch kale (about 9 ounces), deribbed
    and coarsely chopped*

1. Heat oil in large pot over high heat. Add onion, garlic, carrots, celery and rutabaga; sprinkle with salt and pepper and sauté until beginning to soften and brown, about 10 to 11 minutes.

2. Stir in garlic, lentils, and herbes de Provence.

3. Add broth and kale. Bring to boil, stirring to incorporate kale.

4. Reduce heat to medium-low, cover with lid slightly ajar, and simmer until lentils are tender, stirring occasionally, about 20 minutes.

5. Add more broth to thin, if desired. Season with additional salt and pepper, if desired.

THE LENTIL: SMALL BUT MIGHTY!

This small legume—the tiniest of the legume family—packs a powerful nutritional punch.
1 one-cup serving contains:

- Molybdenum—198% of the daily recommended value
- Folate—89.5% of the daily recommended value
- Fiber—62.5% of the daily recommended value
- Tryptophan—50% of the daily recommended value
- Manganese—49% of the daily recommended value
- Iron—36.6% of the daily recommended value
- Protein—35.7% of the daily recommended value
- Phosphorus—35.6% of the daily recommended value
- Copper—25% of the daily recommended value
- Vitamin B12—2% of the daily recommended value
- Potassium—20.8% of the daily recommended value

POTATO SOUP WITH KALE AND CHORIZO

MAKES 6 SERVINGS

I love any kind of potato soup. I find them so warming and comforting. And I love kale! And though my family doesn't eat a lot of animal protein, I do love chorizo used as a flavoring agent, which it is here in this scrumptious recipe. Try this. You'll love it! If you don't have Spanish chorizo, try Portuguese choricua or Calabrese spicy salami. If you want to try a vegan sausage analog here, go right ahead, adding it at the very end of cooking.

5 tablespoons olive oil, divided

1 large onion, chopped (about 2 cups)

8 ounces fully cooked smoked Spanish chorizo or hot Calabrese salami, casing removed and cut into medium dice

2 teaspoons smoked (sweet) paprika

1½ pounds russet potatoes, peeled, cut into large cubes

8 cups low-salt chicken broth

1½ pounds kale, stemmed, torn into small pieces (about 16 cups lightly packed)

Optional garnish: 3 cups croutons (you can use gluten-free croutons if you'd like)

Optional garnish: 2 tablespoons fresh parsley, minced

1. Heat 3 tablespoons oil in large pot over medium heat. Add onion and cook until translucent, about 8 minutes.

2. Add chorizo and paprika, stirring for 1 to 2 minutes.

3. Add potatoes and broth. Increase heat and bring to boil.

4. Add kale and stir until barely softened and soup returns to boil.

5. Reduce heat to low, cover, and simmer for one hour, stirring occasionally.

6. Garnish with optional croutons and/or minced parsley.

WHAT IS CHORIZO?

Chorizo is a cured sausage made from coarsely chopped pork and pork fat, seasoned with smoked pimentón (paprika) and salt. (The Mexican version is uncured and instead of paprika, features dried ground chiles.) Highly flavored, a little bit goes a long way, making it an outstanding flavoring agent and condiment for veggie, bean, or grain dishes.

SAUSAGE: PUTTING IT TO GOOD USE

There are more than 200 types of sausages worldwide—nearly every country has some type of sausage, typically made of chopped animal protein (red meat, poultry, seafood, reptile, or other animal, even soy, grain, legumes, and nuts) and a blend of strong spices. Most of these countries have a range of ways to use these full-flavored foods—I've included a few of these recipes here. I love the idea of using meat as a flavoring agent. What this means: Instead of a big slab of meat, a smaller amount of flavorful animal protein is used to flavor soups, stews, stir-fry, grain dishes—or anything else, really.

KALED-UP SPLIT PEA SOUP

MAKES 4 SERVINGS

As the child of a Dane, I adore split pea soup. It is my absolute favorite, so I've eaten a lot of the stuff in my lifetime. I love it with curry, I love it with fennel, I love it with dill, with caraway, even with nettles and a splash of aquavit. This version surprised me (and yes, I also love it!) with its deep, smoky flavor. It's the sausage (yep, another sausage soup) that gives the soup its deep flavor, though you are welcome to leave the meat out for a vegetarian version.

1   (16-ounce) bag dried green split peas, picked over and rinsed

12 ounces fully cooked smoked pork linguiça or andouille sausages, sliced into ½-inch rounds or cut into a large dice
8   cups (or more) chicken broth
5   Turkish bay leaves
3   to 4 cups coarsely chopped kale
    Salt and pepper to taste

1. In a large pot over medium heat, combine split peas, sausages, eight cups broth, and bay leaves in heavy large pot.

2. Bring to boil over medium-high heat.

3. Add kale, cover, reduce heat to low, and simmer until peas are tender, stirring occasionally, about 25 to 40 minutes.

4. Season to taste with salt and pepper.

LEGUME POINTERS

- Uncooked dry beans can be stored for a year or longer in the unopened plastic bag in which they are sold.
- Once opened, store legumes in an airtight container in a cool, dry place.
- Before preparing, inspect and remove any debris or dirt.
- Dry beans and whole peas need to soak before cooking. Soak in a big pot of cold water overnight, or in hot water for 1 to 4 hours.
- To reduce gas-producing substances, soak longer, then discard the soaking water and use fresh water for cooking.
- Use beans in stews, soups, casseroles, combined with whole grains, in salads, and pureed for dips.
- Stretch meat in meatballs, meatloaf, shepherd's pie, and other dishes by mixing in a cup or two of mashed legumes.
- Lentils and split peas are the "fast foods" in the legume family; they need only about 30 to 40 minutes to cook, no pre-soaking required.
- One cup of dry beans and peas equals about 2½ to 3 cups cooked.
- When drained, a 15-ounce can equals about 1½ cups of beans.

PINTO-BEAN MOLE CHILI

MAKES 6 SERVINGS

I am a chili fanatic. I like it Texas-style. I like it Cincinnati-style and Utah-style and California-style. I like vegetarian and white and black bean and con carne styles. This rich-tasting recipe features a sophisticated mix of spices, for a deeply-flavored, super healthy (spices are rich in antioxidants) dish. Yum, yum, yum!

2   *teaspoons chili powder*
1   *teaspoon chipotle powder*
1   *teaspoon cumin*
1   *teaspoon dried oregano*
½   *teaspoon dried coriander*
Optional: 1 teaspoon epazote
⅛   *to ¼ teaspoon cinnamon*
2   *medium onions, chopped*
2   *tablespoons olive oil*
5   *garlic cloves, minced*
2   *cups butternut or other winter squash, cut into a large dice (you can also use summer squash or sweet potatoes)*
¾   *pound kale, stems, and center ribs discarded and leaves coarsely chopped*
1   *teaspoon agave syrup*
1   *ounce unsweetened chocolate, finely chopped (3 tablespoons)*
1   *(14 ½-ounce) can whole tomatoes in juice*
1¼ *chicken broth*
1   *to 2 tablespoon lime juice*
3   *(15-ounce) cans pinto beans, drained and rinsed*
    Salt to taste
Optional garnishes: salsa, diced avocado, guacamole, chopped scallion or red onion,
sliced radishes, jalapeno slices, rice; chopped cilantro, and/or sour cream

1. In a large pot over medium-high heat, sauté onions, stirring occasionally, until softened. Add garlic and cook, stirring, about one minute.

2. Stir in chili powder, chipotle powder, cumin, oregano, coriander, epazote, and coriander.

3. Stir in squash and kale and cook, covered, 7 to 10 minutes, until squash begins to soften.

4. Stir in agave, chocolate, tomatoes with their juice, broth, and lime juice and simmer, covered, stirring occasionally, until vegetables are tender, about 20 minutes.

5. Stir in beans and simmer another 5 minutes to blend flavors. Season with salt to taste.

PORK PUMPKIN STEW

SERVES 6 TO 8

Pork and pumpkin are a gorgeous taste treat. Add the slightly astringent, green taste of kale and you have a beautiful balance of tastes and textures. You also have a high-nutrient dish, perfecto for a nippy autumn or winter (or even early spring) day. You'll love this!

¼   *cup extra virgin olive oil*
2   *pounds boneless pork shoulder, cut into 1½-inch pieces and patted dry*
2   *onions, chopped*
3   *garlic cloves, minced*
1   *14-ounce can diced tomatoes, including the juice (I love using Muir Glen's fire-roasted diced tomatoes in this recipe)*
1½ *cups chicken broth*

1   *pound red-skinned (boiling) potatoes, cut into 1-inch pieces*
4   *cups kale, deribbed and coarsely chopped*
1   *2-pound sugar pumpkin or other winter squash, de-seeded (reserve the seeds for toasting if desired), peeled, and cut into 1-inch pieces*
    Salt and pepper to taste

1. Preheat oven to 350°F.
2. Add oil to a large heavy, ovenproof pot and set on the stove over medium-high heat. Add pork pieces, a few at a time, browning all sides then transferring pieces with a slotted spoon to a plate or bowl. Continue until all pork pieces are browned. Set pork aside
3. Add chopped onions to the pot and sauté until golden.
4. Add the garlic and sauté for a minute.
5. Add the tomatoes with their juice, the broth, the pork, and any accumulated juices. Bring to a boil and immediately remove from heat.
6. Place pot in oven for one hour.
7. Add potatoes, give the stew a stir, cover and cook for 20 more minutes
8. Add the greens and the pumpkin, give the stew another stir, cover the pot and cook for an additional 20 to 30 minutes, until pumpkin and kale are tender.
9. Season stew with salt and pepper.

PUMPKIN SEEDS: THE ULTIMATE SNACK

My kids' favorite autumn activity is making pumpkin seeds. In the weeks between Halloween and American Thanksgiving, we must roast 10 pumpkins' worth of seeds. It's something I am happy to do with them because not only is it fun to be in the kitchen together, the seeds are deeply nourishing, with vitamins, minerals, antioxidants, omega-3 fatty acids, protein, and fiber. We use the seeds from sugar and other baking-style pumpkins (we like their flavor best), cheese pumpkins, Australian blue Hubbard squash, and kabocha squash. All winter squash seeds can be roasted, but some are tougher to eat than others. Experiment to find your favorite.

If not making a Jack O' Lantern, we simply cut the squash into quarters and throw the innards—goop and all—into a large bowl of cold water. The water softens the bonds between fiber and seeds. We reach into the water and manually separate those seeds that haven't separated naturally. We then place seeds in a single layer on a clean dishtowel to dry. I like to let them dry overnight, but a couple of hours is fine. Some people skip this step and go straight to the roasting, though I find the seeds tougher to chew if you don't first let them air-dry.

To roast seeds, preheat oven to low, about 175°F. In a large bowl, toss seeds with a small splash of tamari and a dash of roasted sesame oil. (You can also try extra virgin olive oil and a dash of salt, virgin coconut oil, and a dash of curry and salt, or any other oil and seasoning combo you can think of.) Lay seeds in a single layer on as many baking sheets as necessary and roast for 15 to 20 minutes, until golden and fragrant.

SALADS

BASIC KALE SALAD
MAKES 6 SERVINGS

This is your basic, build-a-salad recipe. Enjoy it as-is, or throw in a handful of chopped nuts, seeds, or dried fruit. Play around with the oils. Try vinegar (you chose which kind) instead of lemon juice. Vary the spices. Add some minced herbs or your favorite veggie. And so on. Make this every single time your friends come over and soon, you'll be known as of those "I don't need a recipe" kinds of geniuses.

2 *tablespoons extra-virgin olive oil (I like toasted walnut oil in this recipe)*
2 *tablespoons lemon juice*
1 *teaspoon chili powder*
   Salt to taste
2 *bunches kale, deribbed, chopped very, very finely*

1. In a large bowl, whisk together oil, lemon juice, chili powder, and salt.
2. Add kale, toss to combine.
3. Allow to sit for 20 minutes before serving to allow flavors to blend.

BRASSICA SALAD
MAKES 4 SERVINGS

Before I tell you how fun and delicious this healthy recipe is, I want to clear something up: Brassica and Cruciferous are two words

A BETTER KALE SALAD

The key to a great kale salad—in my opinion at least—is to cut the leaves very thin. I like to chiffonade leaves. To do this, derib leaves, stack five to ten of them on top of each other, roll them up into a tube, and cut the tube of leaves into super-thin slices. They are easy to make, pretty, and ready to use in salads, or to sauté or steam.

for the same fabulous family, that large, talented clan that includes kale, collards, cabbage, kohlrabi, Brussels sprouts, and so on. Okay, now for the recipe. This contains two cousins: Kale and Brussels sprouts. (You could use cabbage instead, if you'd like.) It tickles me to use two members of the same family in one dish, especially a dish as tasty as this one. Lacinto kale does well in this recipe.

2 *tablespoons lemon juice*
1 *tablespoon Dijon mustard*
1 *tablespoon minced shallot*
1 *small garlic clove, minced*
   Salt and pepper to taste
   Freshly ground black pepper
1 *large bunch of kale (I prefer Lacinto), deribbed and leaves cut in a chiffonade*
6 *ounces Brussels sprouts (or cabbage), finely sliced*
1 *cup walnuts, toasted and coarsely chopped*
¼ *cup walnut oil (you can also use extra-virgin olive oil), divided*

Optional: ¼ cup finely grated Pecorino

1. In a medium bowl, whisk together lemon juice, mustard, shallot, garlic, a pinch of salt and pepper in a small bowl. Stir to blend. Set aside.

2. Combine kale and Brussels sprouts in a large bowl.

3. Whisk walnut oil into the lemon juice mixture, thoroughly combining. Season with salt and/or pepper, as desired.

4. Drizzle dressing over kale mixture and toss leaves to coat.

5. Add walnuts and pecorino, if using, and combine. Adjust seasonings with salt and/or pepper, as desired.

NUTTY KALE SLAW

MAKES 6 SERVINGS

This may be my favorite kale recipe. I first tasted kale salad at my brother and sister-in-law's house and fell in love with it instantly! Not only does this taste great, it makes me feel wonderful and strong after eating it. This is one of those recipes that people will ask for.

2 *large bunches kale, about 2 pounds, deribbed and cut in a chiffonade*

2 *orange or red bell peppers, cleaned and cut into very fine strips*

1 *large carrot, peeled and shredded (you can use a box grater or a food processor with grater attachment)*

WHY SPROUTS ARE NAMED BRUSSELS

Brussels sprouts and kale are cousins. While it isn't known exactly where these cabbage-like sprouts were first grown, they are believed to have originated in Belgium—they were first mentioned in Brussels in the late 16th century, where they became an important agricultural crop. It was during World War I that this local delicacy caught the attention of European and American soldiers, who named the vegetable after the Belgian city and carried them back to their homelands. And the rest, as they say, is veggie history. As proof of just how far these gorgeous sprouts have wandered from their original home: Today, almost all Brussels sprouts consumed in North America are grown in California.

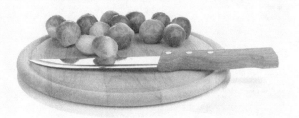

1 cup roasted, salted almonds, pecans, or
  peanuts, divided
Optional: 2 tablespoons cilantro leaves
⅓ cup virgin coconut oil
3 tablespoons apple cider vinegar (you can also
  use lemon juice)
1 tablespoon agave syrup or honey
  Salt and pepper to taste
Optional: Couple shakes of Tabasco or other
  hot sauce

1. In a food processor, pulse together ¼ cup
of the nuts, cilantro, oil, vinegar, agave, salt,
pepper, and hot sauce. Pulse until nuts are
half-way pureed. Set aside

2. In a large bowl, toss together kale, bell
pepper, carrots, and nuts.

3. Using a spatula to get every last drop,
scrape dressing over kale mixture. Toss with
dressing to coat all leaves.

4. Allow dressing to sit for 20 minutes before
serving to blend flavors.

BUTTERNUT SQUASH AND KALE SALAD

MAKES 4 TO 6 SERVINGS

Here it is again—that gorgeous winter squash
and kale combo. It looks beautiful, tastes
wonderful, and is outrageously healthy thanks
to a range of antioxidants, vitamins, minerals,
and fiber. You'll love this cooked salad.

2 bunches kale, deribbed, leaves finely chopped
1 cup chicken broth, divided
1 2-pound butternut squash or other winter
  squash, peeled, deseeded and cut into
  ½-inch cubes

PEANUT POWER

Peanuts have become mired in controversy. For the growing numbers of people allergic to
them, even a small amount of dust or oil can mean anaphylactic shock, a situation where
airways begin to close, cutting off oxygen to an individual. For others, the aflatoxin mold (a
type of fungus) that grows on peanuts can contribute to conditions such as candida, eczema,
and mold allergies. It has also been linked to cancer in laboratory rats, and has been studied as one cause of stunted growth in African populations relying heavily on peanut protein.

Despite all of this, peanuts are a part of American culture, showing up in sandwiches, cook-
ies, smoothies, spread on apples and celery, mixed into ice cream and eaten straight for the jar.
Interestingly, however, peanuts are not originally from North America: They were brought from
South America by Spanish explorers and made popular centuries later by Union and Confeder-
ate soldiers in the American Civil War who needed cheap, portable protein. Also interesting:
Peanuts aren't nuts at all: They are a legume, related to other members of the legume family.

1   red onion, coarsely chopped
4   pitted prunes, dates or ¼ cup raisins, very
    finely chopped
2   tablespoons sherry vinegar

1. In a large pot over medium heat, heat ½ cup of broth and kale. Cook, covered, stirring frequently, until kale is wilted, about 3 to 5 minutes.

2. Add squash and continue cooking, stirring occasionally, until kale and squash are barely fork-tender, about 10 minutes. Remove from heat and allow to cool to room temperature.

3. Meanwhile, in a small saucepan, combine the remaining ½ cup broth, onion, dried fruit, and vinegar in a small saucepan.

4. Bring liquid to a boil, then lower heat and simmer, uncovered, until onion is very tender and liquid is reduced by half, about 7 or 8 minutes.

5. Allow dressing to cool to barely-warm or room temperature. Drizzle over kale-squash mixture and serve room temperature.

DID YOU KNOW…?

Butternut squash is one of the most popular winter squash varieties. This large, pear-shaped squash has a sweet, slightly nutty taste and a smooth, just moist-enough texture. Here are a few reasons to get to know butternuts better:

- Every part of the butternut squash is edible: Its vines, leaves, flowers, flesh, and seeds. In many regions, such as Africa, all parts of the squash are eaten.
- Butternuts belong to the Cucurbitaceae family of field pumpkins, which are believed to have originated in the Central American region
- Butternuts are the most commonly grown winter squash in the Western Hemisphere.
- The butternut plant is monoecious as in pumpkins, and features different male and female flowers that require honeybees for effective pollination.
- Butternuts range in size from less than a pound to over 33 pounds. Most, however, are in the 2- to 5-pound range.
- In Argentina, butternuts are used as livestock food.
- Butternut squash seeds are used as nutritious snack food since they contain 35% to 40% oil and 30% protein. In Argentina, the fruit is also used to feed livestock.
- One cup of cooked butternut squash contains 82 calories and 2 grams of protein.
- It has more vitamin A than pumpkins, providing about 354% of recommended daily allowance.
- It contains plenty of amino acids, antioxidants, B-complex vitamins, iron, zinc, copper, calcium, potassium, phosphorous, and fiber.

KALE QUINOA SALAD

MAKES 4 SERVINGS

Adding grain to this kale salad makes it hearty and rich in protein. If you'd like, substitute the same amount of cooked brown or black or red rice, bulgur, millet, farro, or other favorite grain. You can even add a chopped avocado to the mix.

1 *bunch kale, deribbed and finely chopped*
1 *cup cooked quinoa*
3 *tablespoons prepared vinaigrette or salad dressing*
Optional: 2 tablespoons sunflower seeds, pepitas, or chopped nuts

1. In a large bowl, thoroughly combine all ingredients. Allow to sit for 20 minutes before serving.

FARRO: WHAT IT IS

Those of you who love regional Italian food have probably encountered Farro, popular in Italian soups and risotto-like dishes, it is a chewy, dense, nourishing grain that is grown in central and northern Italy. An ancient parent to wheat, farro was one of the most popular cereal grains in the ancient world. Wild plants were found at an archaeological site carbon dated around 17,000 BCE, in modern-day Israel. References to the plant appear in early Hebrew, Greek, and Latin documents. Today, it remains popular in central and northern Italy, where it is considered a health food of sorts, celebrated for its high protein and fiber content.

BULGUR: WHAT IT IS

Bulgur. Sounds exotic, doesn't it? This Middle Eastern staple is actually made up of wheat kernels that have been steamed, dried, and crushed. It is high in fiber (twice that of brown rice) and protein, low in fat and calories, making it another food that offers bulk and nutrients to fill you up without adding pounds. One thing to keep in mind, however, is because bulgur is made of wheat, it does contain gluten. Celiacs and those on gluten-free diets, you have been warned!

ALL HALLOWS KALE

Among Celtic people, kale is traditionally associated with Halloween, and it is one of the ingredients of colcannon, a dish customarily eaten in Ireland on that day.

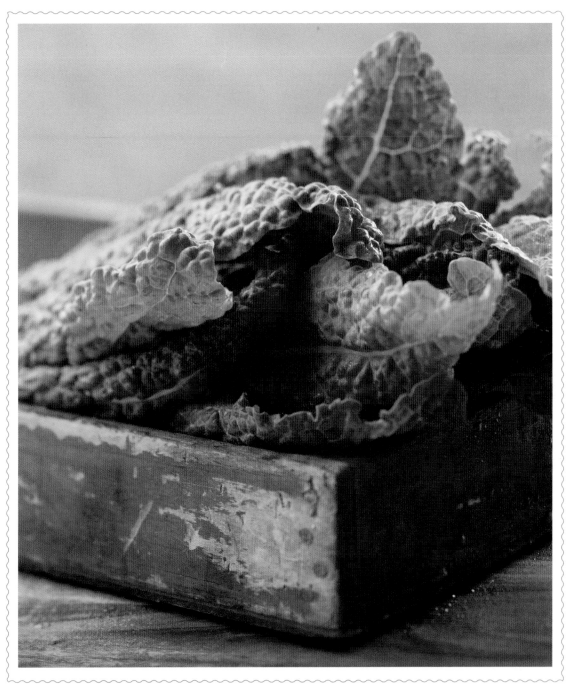

Deeply nourishing, delicious Lacinto kale is also known as Tuscan kale or dinosaur kale.

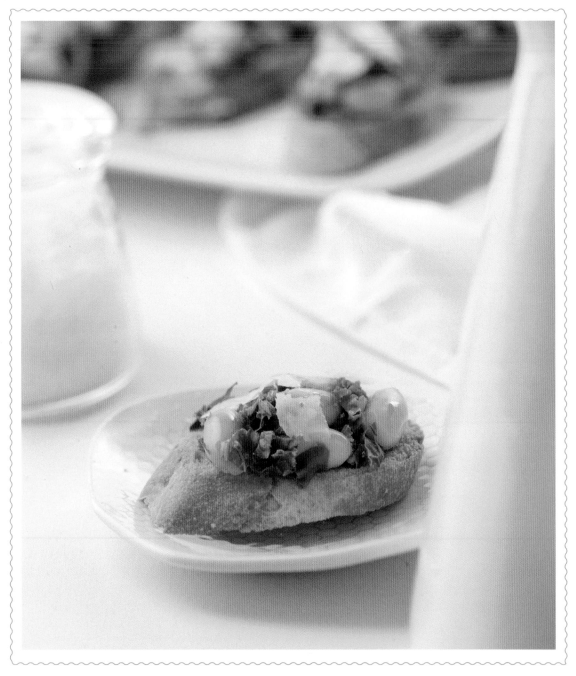

Kale and Bean Bruschetta is the ideal appetizer: Delicious, healthy, easy, and very sophisticated.
Page 114

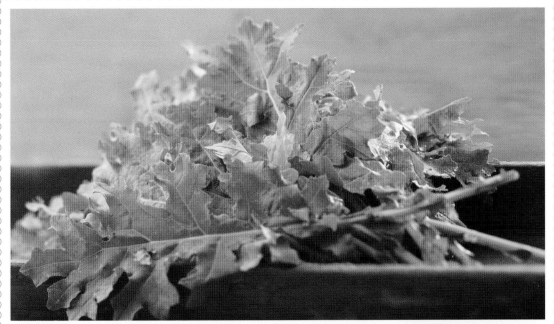

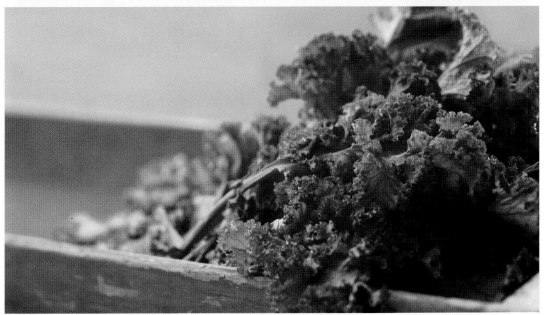

Top: Siberian kale is extremely cold hardy with a rich, almost sweet taste.
Bottom: Beautiful red Russian kale lends a lovely rosey hue to dishes.

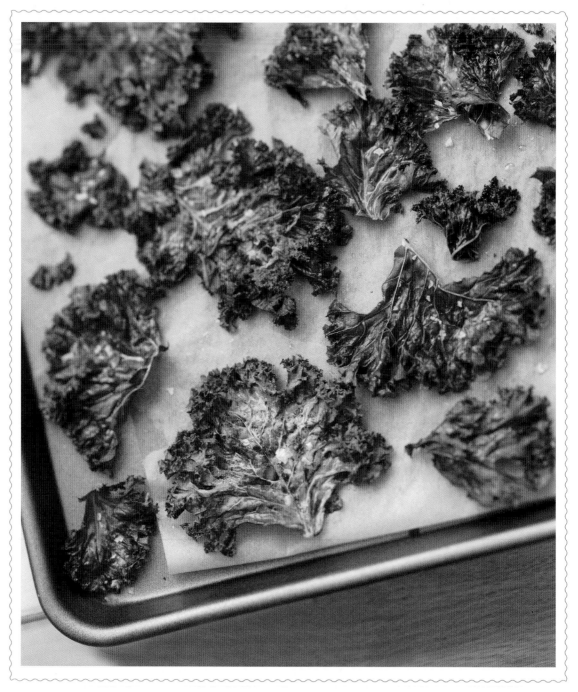

Kale Chips are the ultimate nonguilty pleasure. Crispy, salty, and addictive. Page 106

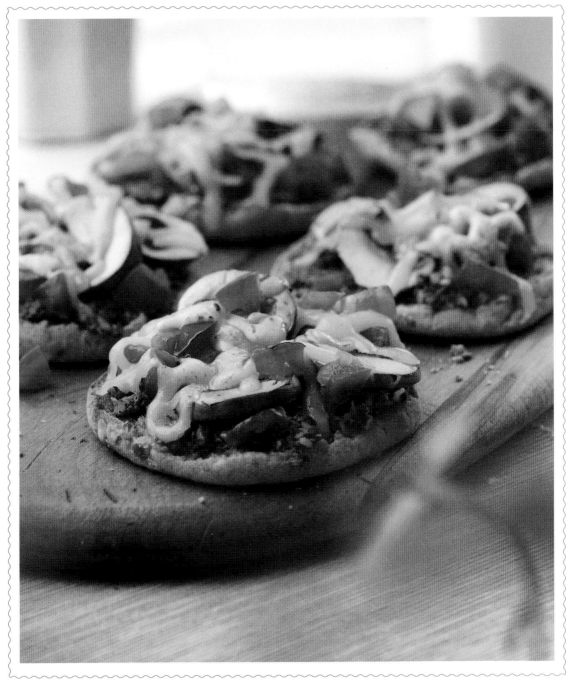

Kale Mini Pizzas are easy, fast, nutritious, and delicious—the perfect afterschool snack! Page 114

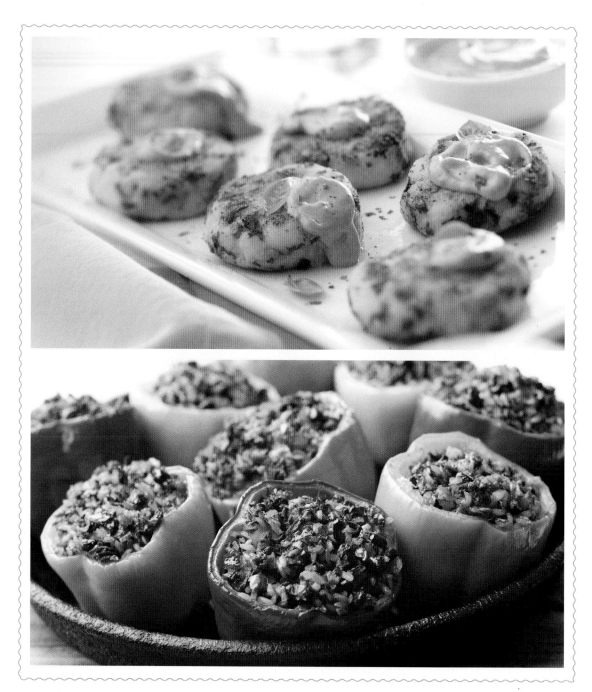

Top: Potato Kale Cakes are a dressy addition to any appetizer tray. Page 140
Bottom: Bell peppers stuffed with Chicken with Kale and Lentil Pilaf. Page 122

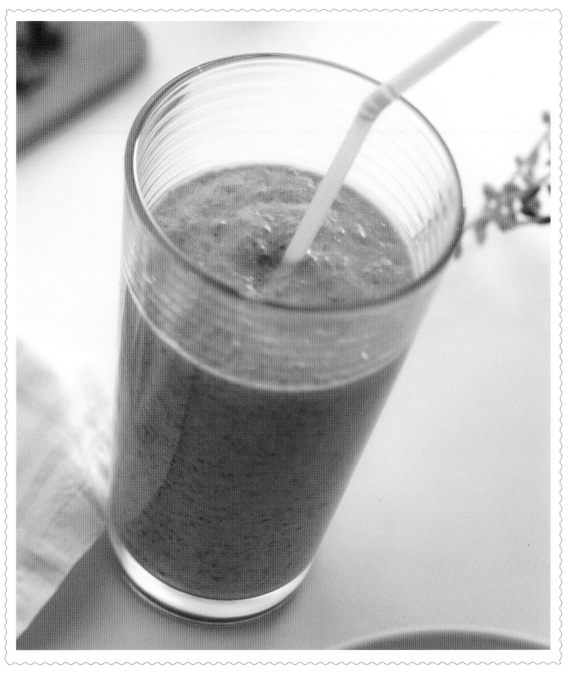

Health in a glass! Superfood Protein Smoothie is ideal as a meal replacement or a quick pick-me-up. Page 40

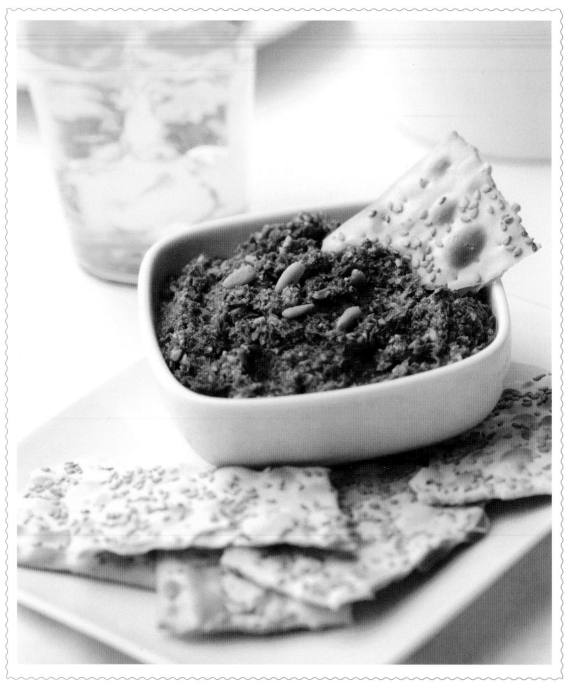

Garlicky Kale and Spinach Dip is a grown-up dip perfect for elegant cocktail parties. Page 119

NUTS-AND-SEED KALE SALAD

MAKES 4 SERVINGS

This is a nutrient-dense salad: Quinoa and the nuts have protein, kale is loaded with iron, avocado boasts brain-boosting fats, and the sesame is rich in calcium.

3 cups cooked quinoa
6 kale leaves, deribbed and finely chopped
½ red or orange pepper, finely chopped
Optional: ½ cup pine nuts
Optional: ¼ cup finely chopped almonds
1 avocado, diced
2 tablespoons lemon juice
2 tablespoons rice vinegar
4 tablespoons roasted sesame oil
1 tablespoon sesame seeds

1. In a large bowl, gently combine quinoa, kale, red pepper, pine nuts, almonds, and avocado.

2. In a small bowl, whisk together lemon juice, rice vinegar, roasted sesame oil, and sesame seeds.

3. Drizzle dressing over kale mixture, gently tossing to combine.

HEALTH BENEFITS OF PINE NUTS

A favorite of gourmet-types, pine nuts—aka pignoli or piñon—add a distinctive flavor and delicate bite to salads, soups, baked goods, grain dishes, and even sauce (pesto anyone?) But foodies aren't the only ones who love pine nuts! Nutritionists, do, too! That's because the small seeds (yes, they are actually pine tree seeds, which nestle in the crevices of pine cones) are rich in vitamins, antioxidants, and minerals and packed with numerous health promoting phyto-chemicals.

Pine nuts are an excellent source of vitamin E, with about 9.33 mg—or about 62 percent of the recommended daily allowance—per 100-gram serving. Vitamin E is a powerful antioxidant. Pine nuts are an excellent source of the B-complex group of vitamins such as thiamin, riboflavin, niacin, pantothenic acid, vitamin B-6 (pyridoxine), and folates. These vitamins help maintain a healthy nervous system. Pine nuts also boast essential minerals like potassium, calcium, iron, magnesium, zinc, and selenium. Plus: they are one of the richest sources of the mineral manganese around, boasting 8.802 mg of manganese—about 383 percent of the daily recommended intake—per 100-gram serving. Manganese happens to be essential in helping the body develop resistance against infectious agents and in obliterating harmful oxygen free radicals.

SESAME FACTS

- Sesame seeds have been grown in tropical regions throughout the world since prehistoric times.
- "Open sesame"—the famous phrase from the *Arabian Nights*—reflects the distinguishing feature of the sesame seed pod, which bursts open when it reaches maturity.
- The scientific name for sesame seeds is *Sesamun indicum*.
- Sesame seeds were one of the first crops processed for oil as well as one of the earliest condiments.
- Foods made with sesame seeds include tahini, halvah, hummus, and baba ganous.
- The seeds were thought to have first originated in India, where they symbolized immortality. From India, sesame seeds were introduced throughout the Middle East.
- Most of the sesame seeds we eat are grown in India, China, and Mexico, the three largest commercial producers of the seeds.
- Sesame seeds are a very good source of manganese, copper, calcium, magnesium, iron, phosphorus, vitamin B1, zinc, and dietary fiber.
- Sesame seeds contain two special lingnans called *sesamin* and *sesamolin*, both of which have been shown to have a cholesterol-lowering effect in humans.

KALE WALDORF SALAD

MAKES 4 SERVINGS

This yummy salad is a revved up version of the well-loved classic. Though it uses most of the same ingredients as the original, I've got to admit it tastes nothing like it. (Not to disparage the first Waldorf salad, but this version is also way more nutritious, thanks to nutrient-packed kale.) Enjoy!

4   *cups Lacinto kale, deribbed and finely chopped*
1   *large tangy, hard apple, (such as Fuji or Honey-crisp), cut into a medium dice and divided*
1   *cup thinly sliced celery*
¾   *cup plus ¼ cup toasted walnuts, chopped*
¼   *cup plus 2 tablespoons raisins, divided*
2   *tablespoons Dijon mustard*
1   *tablespoon walnut oil*
2   *tablespoons water*
1   *tablespoon red wine vinegar*
    Salt and pepper to taste

1. In a large bowl, combine kale, half the apple, celery, ¾ cup of the walnuts, and ¼ cup of the raisins. Toss to combine.

2. In the bowl of a food processor or in a high-power blender, add ¼ cup walnuts, 2 tablespoons raisins, mustard, walnut oil, water, vinegar, salt, and pepper. Purée until well combined and slightly thick, adding additional water if necessary to keep a "dressing-like" consistency.

3. Drizzle dressing over kale mixture, tossing gently to combine.

SANDWICHES

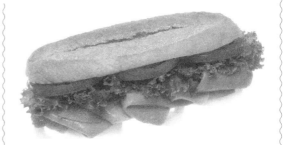

SPICY KALE-CHEESE SANDWICH

MAKES 4 SERVINGS

This yummy sandwich adds a fresh (and healthy) twist on the everyday grilled cheese. I love this with a bowl of soup!

1 *cup grated mild cheese, such as Monterey Jack*
1 *cup finely chopped kale*
1 *garlic clove, minced*
¼ *to ½ teaspoon Tabasco or other hot sauce*
  Salt and pepper to taste
8 *slices whole grain bread*
3 *tablespoons or more Dijon or other spicy mustard*
2 *tablespoons or more softened butter, divided*

1. In a large bowl, mix together cheese, kale, garlic, hot sauce and salt and pepper. Set aside.
2. Spread the inside of each piece of bread with mustard.
3. Create four sandwiches by topping four slices of bread with ¼ cup filling, then topping with remaining bread slices.
4. Butter the outsides of all bread.
5. Place a large skillet over medium-high heat. Place sandwiches in skillet and cook until one side is brown.
6. Turn sandwiches. Cook until second side is brown and cheese has melted.

GOOD KARMA KALE SANDWICH

MAKES 1 SERVING

It seems almost wrong to me to give you recipes for sandwiches. In my world, sandwiches are ad hoc things, stacked together with whatever sounds good at the moment, coupled with whatever we have in the fridge. It's from that creative yet practical place, that this Good Karma Sandwich comes from! Feel free to change it up in any way that appeals to you!

2 *tablespoons hummus or refried beans or white bean dip*
2 *pieces whole grain bread*
1 *thin slice red onion*
¼ *cup leftover kale salad or cooked kale dressed with 2 teaspoons of your favorite dressing*

1. Toast bread until golden.
2. Spread toasted bread with hummus.
3. Cover one slice of bread with leftover kale salad and red onion. Top with remaining piece of toasted bread.

KALE IN SCOTLAND

Kale was grown as a staple crop in the Scottish Islands due to its extreme hardiness, and was given protection from the elements in purpose-built kale yards. Indeed, almost every house had a kale yard and preserved kale in barrels of salt, similar to sauerkraut in Germany. They also fed it to livestock through the winter. Kale continued to be extremely important until potatoes came to the Islands towards the end of the 18th century.

VINEGAR ON GREENS?

When I was growing up, any time we had kale or spinach with dinner, my mom would plunk down a bottle of vinegar next to the serving dish. For us, the vinegar was a liter of store brand apple cider vinegar. But from what I now know, my family wasn't the only one who served their greens with vinegar; this is common practice the world over.

But why? Taste, for one. Vinegar adds spark and tang to bitter greens. But perhaps a more important reason, one my own mother did not know about, is that vinegar makes the calcium in dark leafy greens more bioavailable. Let me explain: While these greens are naturally high in calcium, they contain a compound that inhibits the body's ability to absorb the mineral. Vinegar deactivates these compounds, allowing the body to benefit from every drop of this bone-building mineral.

CARAMELIZED SHALLOT-KALE-PROSCIUTTO SANDWICH

MAKES 2 SERVINGS

Can a sandwich be elegant? (Particularly a sandwich that contains kale?) I say yes! Try this recipe and see for yourself.

1   *tablespoon extra virgin olive oil*
2   *shallots, sliced thin*
1   *garlic clove, coarsely chopped*
½   *cup fresh kale, cut into 1- to 2-inch pieces*
4   *slices prosciutto*
4   *ounces goat cheese*
4   *slices sourdough sandwich bread*
    Salt and pepper to taste

1. Heat olive oil in a medium skillet over medium-low heat. Add the shallot and garlic to the pan and sauté, stirring often, until brown, soft and buttery in texture, about 12 minutes. (Add more oil or a teaspoon or more of water if shallots begin to stick.)
2. Add the kale to the pan and sauté until wilted and softened. Season with salt and pepper.
3. Toast bread.
4. Spread the inside of each piece of toasted bread with goat cheese.
5. Divide the prosciutto between the sandwiches, then place shallot-kale mixture atop prosciutto.
6. Top with remaining slices of bread.

TURKEY ORCHARD SANDWICH

MAKES 1 SERVING

This is a fun, sweet-savory sandwich that's a bit different than your everyday lunch. It reminds me of Thanksgiving.

2   *slices whole grain bread*
½   *tablespoon Dijon mustard*
Optional: 2 tablespoons cranberry sauce
3   *to 4 ounces sliced turkey breast (sliced turkey deli meat is fine)*
1   *slightly firm Bosc pear or Asian pear, sliced into very thin slices*
2   *raw kale leaves*

1. Spread inside of bread with mustard.
2. If using, spread cranberry sauce over the mustard.
3. Layer turkey, pear slices, and kale leaves on top of one slice of bread.
4. Top with remaining bread slice.

KALE FOR VICTORY!

During World War II, citizens of the UK were encouraged by their government to grow kale as part of the country's Dig for Victory campaign. Why kale? It is easy to grow and provides important nutrients missing during the wartime diet because of rationing.

PEARS: DID YOU KNOW...?

- One pear contains 22% of your daily recommended allowance of fiber, 12.4% of vitamin C, and 10% of vitamin K.
- The gritty fiber in pears has been found to bind to cancer-causing toxins and chemicals in the colon, protecting it from contact with these poisons.
- Pears are rich in antioxidant carotenoids such as lutein, and zeaxanthins and flavonols such as querticin and kaempferol, all of which have been shown to have antioxidant as well as anti-inflammatory benefits.
- Pears have been associated with lowered risk of several common chronic diseases caused by chronic inflammation and excessive oxidative stress, including cardiovascular disease and diabetes.
- Pears contain some copper, iron, potassium, manganese, and magnesium, as well as B-complex vitamins.
- Herbalists suggest using pears to treat colitis, chronic gallbladder disorders, arthritis, and gout.

CHICKPEA AND KALE SANDWICH SPREAD OR SALAD

MAKES 4 SERVINGS

I love the idea of stuffing pita bread with a hearty, delicious filling—it's my favorite type of grab-and-go sandwich! You must try this delicious recipe—it just may replace your current hummus sandwich. I like to add slices of cucumber and a shredded carrot for a bright, fresh taste.

4   *medium kale leaves, deribbed*
1   *tablespoon yellow mustard*
2   *tablespoons extra virgin olive oil*
1   *to 2 tablespoons fresh dill leaves*
1   *scallions, white and light green portion*
1   *to 2 tablespoons lemon juice or rice vinegar,*
     to taste
½   *teaspoon curry powder*
½   *teaspoon ground cumin*
     Freshly ground pepper to taste
1   *(15- to 16-ounce) can chickpeas,*
     drained and rinsed (you can also use
     cannellini beans)

1. In a food processor, add all ingredients except chickpea and avocado. Pulse until mixture is smooth and thoroughly blended.

2. Add chickpeas and optional avocado and pulse just to chop and slightly blend. You want this mixture chunky.

3. Serve in a pita, on crackers, between slices of bread or as a salad.

WHAT IS DILL?

Part of the Umbellifarae family, which includes carrots and parsley, dill is a popular culinary plant. Both its leaves and seeds are used. The herb is popular in Scandinavian, northern Russian, and Polish cooking. The Scandinavians use so much of the stuff that they gave the plant the name we now use: "Dill" comes from the old Norse word *dilla* which means "to lull." This name reflects dill's traditional uses as both a carminative stomach soother and an insomnia reliever.

WHEN IN ROME...

The chickpea held a place of honor in food-loving ancient Rome. In fact, the legume was so valued, that the leader Cicero proudly claimed his name derived from *cicer*, the Latin term for chickpea. One of Cicero's ancestors was named Cicero because he had a wart on his nose that looked like a chickpea.

A BEAN BY ANY OTHER NAME...

A chickpea by any other name would be—yep, a chickpea! This member of the pea family is called *garbanzo* in Spanish-speaking countries, *ceci* in Italy, *chiche* in French.

Whatever you call them, they are the world's most widely-consumed legume. Probably because they taste so great, are easy to cook, and are terrifically versatile. They are also incredibly nutrient-dense, boasting protein, calcium, iron, and phosphorous.

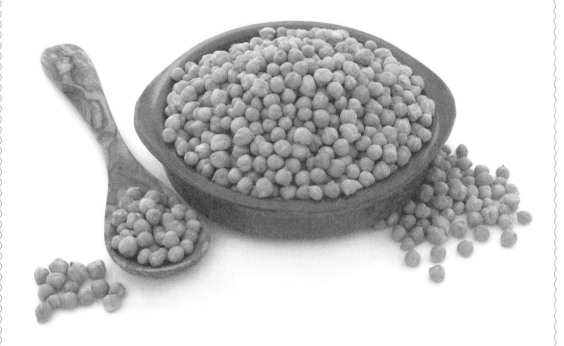

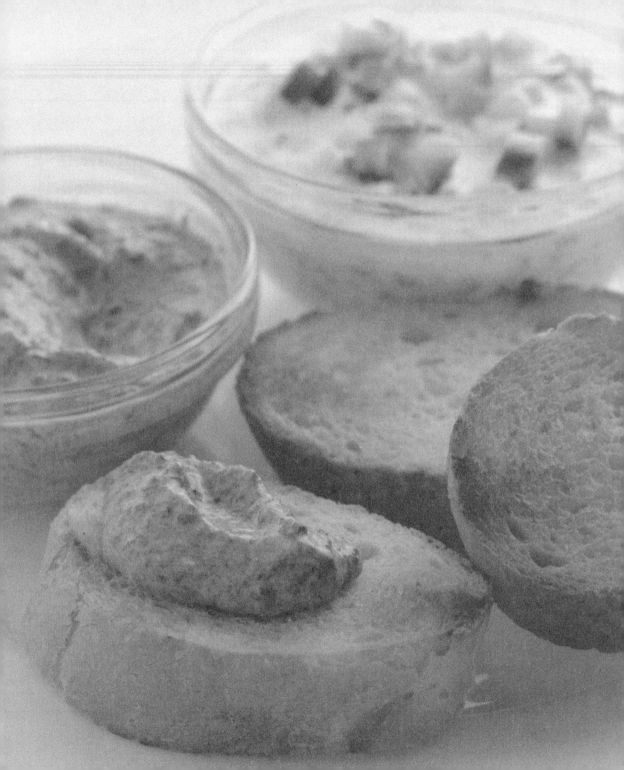

CHAPTER 6

SMALL BITES:
KALE APPETIZERS AND SNACKS

Sometimes you just want a little something. A snack. Or something fancy before a dinner party so you can show off your ingenious culinary skills. Then there are the times your kids come home from school or soccer practice absolutely famished and you want something yummy and healthy to offer them.

Instead of something out of a bag, think kale. Yes, kale! Kale is so versatile that it lends itself to a wide variety of appetizers, sandwiches, dips, and more. Get creative. Try the recipes in this section and then get improvising. I'm sure you'll come up with all kinds of yummy kale munchies.

KALE CHIPS AND CRACKERS

KALE CRACKERS

MAKES 2 TO 4 SERVINGS

Once you've mastered kale chips, you may want to try your hand at something a bit more substantial, like these fun and very healthy crackers! We love them with a bit of hummus.

6   leaves of Lacinto kale, deribbed
⅔   cup ground almonds or mixture of walnuts, pecans, and almonds
¼   cup sesame seeds
2   tablespoons chia seed
¼   cup nutritional yeast
½   teaspoon salt
    Dash pepper
1   teaspoon curry powder, chili powder, chipotle powder, or other favorite spice

1. Preheat oven to 250°F.
2. Line a baking sheet with parchment or aluminum foil.
3. Add kale to the bowl of a food processor. Pulse until ground into a paste.
4. Add remaining ingredients and pulse until combined.
5. Using a silicone spatula, spread mixture onto prepared baking sheet. Score into crackers (make them on the small size; the crackers break easily when too large).
6. Bake for 40 to 45 minutes.

BAKED KALE CHIPS

SERVES 4

These are a low calorie nutritious snack. Like potato chips, you cannot stop at just eating one. They are great for parties and a good conversation topic. They're also loaded with vitamins, minerals, phytonutrients, and fiber.

1 *bunch kale*
1 *tablespoon olive oil*
1 *teaspoon seasoned salt*

1. Preheat an oven to 350° F.
2. Line a non-insulated cookie sheet with parchment paper.
3. With a knife or kitchen shears carefully remove the leaves from the thick stems and tear into bite size pieces. Wash and thoroughly dry kale with a salad spinner. Drizzle the kale with olive oil and sprinkle with seasoning salt.
4. Bake until the edges brown but are not burnt, 10 to 15 minutes.

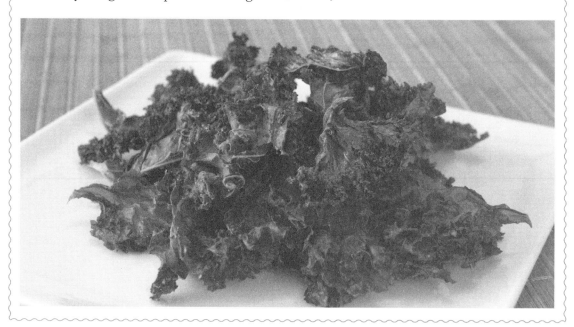

SALT AND VINEGAR KALE CHIPS

MAKES 4 SERVINGS

Crispy baked kale is seasoned with vinegar and salt in this snack recipe. It's a great healthy replacement to salt and vinegar chips.

1   bunch kale
1   tablespoon extra-virgin olive oil, divided
1   tablespoon sherry vinegar
1   pinch sea salt, to taste

1. Preheat an oven to 300°F (150°C).
2. Cut away inner ribs from each kale leaf and discard; tear the leaves into pieces of uniform size. (I made my pieces about the size of a small potato chip.) Wash torn kale pieces and spin dry in a salad spinner or dry with paper towels until they're very dry.
3. Put the kale pieces into a large resealable bag (or use a bowl if you don't mind getting your hands oily). Add about half the olive oil; seal and squeeze the bag so the oil gets distributed evenly on the kale pieces. Add the remaining oil and squeeze the bag more, until all kale pieces are evenly coated with oil and slightly "massaged."
4. Sprinkle the vinegar over the kale leaves, reseal the bag, and shake to spread the vinegar evenly over the leaves. Spread the leaves evenly onto a baking sheet.
5. Roast in the preheated oven until mostly crisp, about 35 minutes. Season with salt and serve immediately.

KALE AND FRUIT SNACKS

KALE CACAO ENERGY TRUFFLES

MAKES 16 TO 18 TRUFFLES

Sometimes you want something rich, chewy. This chocolate-based recipe is a great, healthy, yummy way to take care of yourself and indulge in the sweetness you crave.

1   cup cashews
¼   cup rice or hemp or legume-based protein
     powder, vanilla flavored or unflavored
¼   cup finely chopped kale leaves
½   cup pitted dates, packed
½   cup pitted prunes, packed (or you can omit
     the prunes and use 1 cup of dates)
2   tablespoons agave nectar
     Splash vanilla
     Dash salt
     Dash cinnamon
¼   cup cacao nibs

1. In the bowl of a food processor, add cashews and hemp protein. Pulse until mixture is coarse.
2. Add the kale, dates, and prunes and pulse until uniformly ground and it sticks together easily.
3. Add the agave, vanilla, salt, and cinnamon and pulse a few more times, until combined.

4. Add the cacao nibs and pulse until mixture is combined.

5. Refrigerate mixture for an hour or more.

6. Shape mixture into 1-inch balls, storing in the refrigerator.

HEALTH BENEFITS OF DATES

- Dates contain high amounts of dietary fiber, which can help with everything from cholesterol levels to digestion.
- The fruit contains flavonoid antioxidants that boast anti-inflammatory properties, while simultaneously strengthening the immune system and helping with healthy blood clotting.
- Dates contain vitamins A, B-complex, and K.
- The fruit is rich in the minerals iron, potassium, calcium, manganese, copper, and magnesium.

KALE CHEESE DATES

MAKES 6 TO SERVINGS

This simple appetizer needs only dates, kale, and almonds (and toothpicks) to prepare—and is sure to be a crowd-pleaser with a lovely mixture of sweet and savory.

¼ cup cooked, steamed, or blanched kale, squeezed dry

1 (8-ounce) brick or tub of cream cheese (can be non-dairy cream cheese)

1 pound whole pitted dates

1. Place kale and cheese in the bowl of a food processor. Pulse or mix until just blended. You want flecks of kale spread throughout the cream cheese.

2. Split the dates in half lengthwise.

3. Spoon a bit of kale-cream cheese mixture into the cavity of each date.

4. Refrigerate finished dates for 20 minutes or more before serving.

KALE GRANOLA BARS

MAKES ABOUT 18 BARS

Who doesn't love granola bars? They are crunchy, sweet, hearty, filling—and in this recipe, they also contain nutrient-dense kale!

2 cups old-fashioned oats

¼ cooked or steamed kale, squeezed dry and finely chopped

½ cup raisins or other dried fruit (coarsely chopped)

½ cup toasted walnuts or pecans, toasted

1 teaspoon ground cinnamon

½ teaspoon ground ginger or fresh grated ginger

6 tablespoons virgin coconut oil

⅓ cup packed dark brown sugar

3 tablespoons honey

1. Preheat oven to 350°F.

2. Line 9-inch square baking pan with foil, allowing foil to extend over sides. Grease foil.

3. In a large bowl, stir together oats, kale, raisins, walnuts, cinnamon, and ginger.

DATES: DID YOU KNOW...?

- Dates originated around the Persian Gulf.
- There is archaeological evidence of date cultivation in the area that is now western Pakistan from around 7,000 BCE.
- Ancient Egyptians made dates into wine.
- In later times, traders from the Middle East and Africa introduced dates to Spain. It was the Spaniards who, in turn, introduced dates to Mexico and California in 1765.
- Dates are naturally pollinated by the wind, but in many modern commercial orchards, farmers pollinate the trees manually. This is done by skilled "pollinators" standing on ladders.
- In the Sahara, dried dates are often fed to camels, horses, and dogs.
- Young date leaves are cooked and eaten as a vegetable, as is the terminal bud or heart, though its removal kills the palm.
- In times of famine, date seeds are often ground into a meal and mixed with flour that is used to make daily bread.
- The date tree has male and female flowers. The female blooms are edible and often used in salads or ground with dried fish to make a condiment.
- In India and Pakistan, North Africa, Ghana, and Côte d'Ivoire, date palms are tapped for the sweet sap, which is converted into palm sugar called jaggery or gur. This sap is also used as a molasses-like syrup or brewed into alcoholic beverages.
- To reduce the potency of their hand-crafted beer, Nigerians often mix in dates (and peppers).
- In North Africa, mature date leaves are used to make huts. They are also used in many cultures to create mats, screens, baskets, and fans.
- The wood from date palm trees is light and durable and is used for construction or burned as fuel.
- When Muslims break fast in the evening meal of Ramadan, it is traditional to eat a date first.
- Ground date seeds are also used as an additive to coffee.
- Another use for ground date seeds: As animal feed.

4. In a medium saucepan over medium heat, combine coconut oil, sugar, and honey. Stir until mixture is smooth and begins to boil.

5. Pour oil mixture over oat mixture. Stir until oat mixture is well coated.

6. Using a silicone spatula, transfer batter to prepared pan. Press down firmly on mixture.

7. Bake until top is golden, about 30 minutes.

8. Allow to cool before using the foil as a handle and removing the bars out of the pan.

9. Place the granola bar onto a flat surface. Using a very sharp knife, cut into 18 bars. (If they crumble as you cut them, you may need to allow them to cool further.)

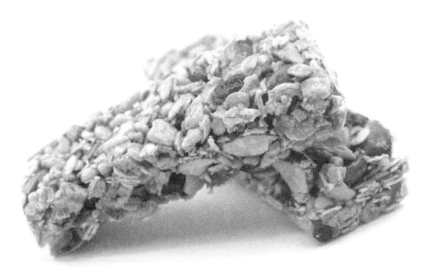

YUMMY THINGS TO DO WITH GINGER

- Spiced-up grains: Grate a bit of ginger into your next pot of millet, rice, quinoa, or other grain. Great served with curries and stir-fries.
- Ginger lemonade: Simply combine freshly grated ginger, lemon juice, and either cane juice or honey and water.
- Perk up bottled salad dressing or a simple homemade vinaigrette with grated ginger.
- Add dry powdered or grated fresh ginger to pureed sweet potatoes. A squirt of lemon juice is a yummy addition.
- Add zing to your next fruit salad with by adding some grated ginger.
- Dress up sautéed veggies by tossing in a half-teaspoon of minced fresh ginger.

SAVORIES

KALE AND GORGONZOLA SWIRLS

MAKES 24 SERVINGS

Serve these scrumptious savory bites at a party and watch them disappear. They have a grown-up, sophisticated flavor—and yet their cheesiness will appeal to the child in each of us.

1   *piece frozen puff pastry, thawed*
1   *bunch blanched kale, deribbed, squeezed dry and finely chopped*
2   *cloves garlic, minced*
2   *tablespoons butter*
1   *egg, beaten in a small bowl with one tablespoon water*
⅓   *cups Gorgonzola cheese, crumbled*
¼   *cups grated Parmesan cheese*

1. Preheat oven to 400°F.
2. Prepare a baking sheet with parchment paper or aluminum foil.
3. Thaw puff pastry according to package directions.
4. Melt butter in a large pot over medium-high heat. Add garlic and sauté for 1 minute.
5. Add kale and sauté tender, about 2 to 3 minutes. Transfer to a bowl to cool.
6. Roll out thawed puff pastry on a floured surface to create a 13-inch square.
7. Brush puff pastry with half of egg-water mixture.

8. Spread kale mixture over entire surface of puff pastry.
9. Sprinkle cheeses evenly over the kale mixture.
10. Roll the puff pastry along the longest side, rolling tightly. When finished, pinch the roll together.
11. Using a sharp, serrated knife, slice the roll into ½-inch slices. (For you bakers out there, use the same process you'd use to make cinnamon rolls.)
12. Place slices at a time onto baking sheet lined with parchment paper. Bake for 15 minutes or until edges are golden. Serve immediately.

DOES KALE HAVE AN IDEAL COOKING TIME?

The noted herbalist, Susun Weed, maintains that kale offers the most nutrition when cooked for 40 minutes—though scientists have yet to study this.

KALE AS INSULT

Early in the 20th century, Kailyard (kale field) was a disparaging term used to describe a school of Scottish writers, including *Peter Pan* author J. M. Barrie, whose writing featured sentimental nostalgia for rural Scottish life.

CHICKEN AND KALE HAND PIES

MAKES 6 SERVINGS

These pies would also be delicious with spinach or Swiss chard in place of the kale. Or, make a vegetarian version with sautéed mushrooms instead of the chicken. You could even change things up further by using ground beef or pork or sausage in place of the poultry. Get creative!

2   *discs pie dough, either homemade or purchased*
2   *tablespoons all-purpose flour, plus, if needed, more for rolling*
1   *tablespoon unsalted butter*
1   *leek (white and light-green parts only), halved lengthwise, cut crosswise ¼-inch thick, and rinsed well*
1   *small bunch Lacinto kale, deribbed and coarsely chopped*
1   *teaspoon fresh thyme leaves*
¼   *teaspoon dried sage*
    Salt, to taste
    Pepper, to taste
1   *cup chicken broth*
1   *cup cooked chicken or turkey, shredded into bite-size pieces (about 5 ounces)*
1   *large egg, lightly beaten*

1. Preheat oven to 425°F.
2. Prepare two baking sheets with parchment or aluminum foil.
3. On a cool surface, roll out one disc of pie dough to a 14-inch round. Dust with flour first if needed to prevent sticking. With a knife or biscuit cutter, cut out six 4¼-inch circles, re-rolling dough just once if necessary. Note: These are the smaller rounds.
4. Transfer cut dough and transfer, on parchment, to a baking sheet. Repeat with remaining dough, cutting out six larger, 4½-inch rounds.
5. Place sheet in the refrigerator until ready to use.
6. In a large skillet over medium-high heat, melt butter. Add leek and sauté until soft, about 3 minutes.
7. Add kale, thyme, salt, and pepper, to the skillet and sauté until kale wilts, about 3 to 5 minutes.
8. Sprinkle flour over mixture. Stir to combine. Add broth and bring to a boil. Cook, stirring often, until mixture thickens, about 2 minutes.
9. Transfer to a medium bowl, season with more salt and pepper if desired, and stir in chicken. Let cool slightly.
10. Remove rounds from refrigerator.
11. Place a rounded ¼ cup chicken mixture on each of the smaller dough rounds, leaving a ½-inch border. Brush edges with egg and top with larger dough rounds; using fingers, press edges firmly to seal.
12. Cut a small vent in each pie. Bake until browned and crisp, 30 minutes, rotating sheet halfway through.

13. Let cool slightly on sheets that have been set on a wire rack. Serve warm or at room temperature.

THYME FOR ORAL HEALTH

Because of its antiseptic, antifungal, and antibacterial properties, herbalists have traditionally used thyme (pronounced "time") as a rinse, gargle, and mouthwash to help cure gum conditions, sore throats, oral burns (such as the dreaded pizza mouth), bad breath, and cavities.

BAKED FETA WITH KALE PESTO ON BAGUETTE

MAKES 8 SERVINGS

A little of this flavorful combo goes a long way, making it a true crowd-pleaser. For a gluten-free option, serve on gluten-free toasts or crackers.

1 *8-ounce piece of mild feta cheese, drained and patted dry*
2 *tablespoons extra-virgin olive oil*
½ *teaspoons dried rosemary*
½ *teaspoon dried basil*
½ *teaspoon dried parsley*
¼ *teaspoon black pepper*
1 *bunch kale, deribbed*
⅓ *cup toasted walnuts*
1 *or 2 garlic cloves*

2 *tablespoons lemon juice*
1 *sourdough or other baguette, thinly sliced*

1. Preheat oven to 400°F.

2. Place feta in a small oiled casserole dish with oil on top. Bake until warm throughout, about 20 minutes.

3. Meanwhile, pulse kale, rosemary, basil, parsley, pepper, walnuts, and garlic in a food processor until finely chopped.

4. With motor running, drizzle in oil and lemon juice to make a pesto. Spoon pesto around feta and bake 5 minutes more.

5. Serve with baguette slices.

ROSEMARY BENEFITS

Rosemary contains a host of vitamins and minerals, including vitamins A, B-complex, and C, as well as minerals potassium, calcium, iron, manganese, copper, and magnesium. It also contains rosmarinic acid, a natural polyphenolic antioxidant that boasts anti-bacterial, anti-inflammatory, and anti-oxidant functions. For the record, the herbs sage, peppermint, oregano, and thyme also contain rosmarinic acid.

KALE MINI PIZZAS

MAKES 4 SERVINGS

Kale is blended into sauce and used to top these yummy treats. Use whatever base you have on hand, from English muffins to pita breads. As you've probably already guessed, kids love these!

1   *cups cooked or steamed kale, squeezed dry and coarsely chopped*
2   *cup marinara or prepared pasta sauce*
¼   *teaspoon freshly ground black pepper*
4   *whole-grain English muffins, split (you can also use tortillas, pitas breads, or individual pizza crusts)*
½   *cup or more shredded part-skim mozzarella cheese*
Optional toppings: sliced olives, mushrooms, peppers, onions, pepperoni, or anything else that sounds appealing

1. Preheat oven to 425°F.
2. Place kale and marinara sauce in a food processor. Pulse until blended. You can leave the kale visible or, for picky eaters, you can puree the sauce until the kale is smooth.

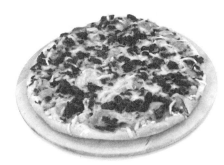

3. Arrange muffin halves on a large baking sheet. Spread sauce on muffins.
4. Top muffins with cheese and optional toppings.
5. Bake until muffins are crisp and cheese is melted, 20 to 25 minutes.

KALE AND BEAN BRUSCHETTA

MAKES 12 SERVINGS

This easy bruschetta is fun, fast, and insanely delicious. It's a terrific option for the vegetarians in your midst. Make it vegan by omitting the cheese. You can even make it gluten-free by serving this on gluten-free toast or on rice crackers.

1   *garlic clove, cut in half*
1   *cups cooked cannellini beans*
½   *cups cooked or steamed kale, squeezed dry and finely chopped*
    Salt, to taste
    Pepper, to taste
Optional: Parmesan cheese shavings
1   *long baguette, sliced into 12 half-inch-thick slices and toasted*

1. In a large bowl, mix beans and kale. Season with salt and pepper.
2. Rub cut side of garlic on toasts.
3. Spoon bean-kale mixture onto toasts. Top with Parmesan shavings if desired.

PIZZA TRIVIA

- In 1987, October was named National Pizza Month.
- Americans eat approximately 350 slices of pizza per second.
- Each man, woman, and child in America eats an average of 46 slices (23 pounds) of pizza a year.
- Approximately 3 billion pizzas are sold in the U.S. each year.
- According to a recent Gallup Poll, kids between the ages of 3 to 11 prefer pizza to all other food groups for lunch and dinner.
- Basic pizza most likely began in prehistoric times, with bread cooked on flat, hot stones.
- Pizza as we know it could not have evolved until the late 1600s when Old World Europeans overcame their fear of tomatoes. Native to Peru and Ecuador, tomatoes came to Europe in the 1500s, carried back by Conquistadors to Spain; tomatoes were believed to be poisonous. It wasn't until the late 1600s that Europeans began to eat the tomato.
- Modern pizza was born in 1889 when Queen Margherita Teresa Giovanni, the consort of Umberto I, king of Italy, visited Naples. Don Raffaele Esposito, who owned a tavern-like place called Pietro Il Pizzaiolo, was asked to prepare a special dish in honor of the Queen's visit. Esposito developed a pizza featuring tomatoes, mozzarella cheese and basil, which mimicked the colors of the Italian flag. He named it the Margherita Pizza, after the guest of honor.
- In 1905, Gennaro Lombardi opened Lombardi's Pizzeria Napoletana, at 53½ Spring Street in New York City. This was the first licensed pizzeria in the United States.
- Pizza became an international food when World War II servicemen returned from Italy, abuzz about "that delicious Italian pizza."
- Pepperoni is America's favorite topping (36 percent of all pizza orders); we eat approximately 251,770,000 pounds per year.
- Anchovies are American's least favorite pizza topping.
- Women are twice as likely as men to order vegetable toppings on their pizza.
- Three of the top 10 weeks of pizza consumption occur in January. More pizza is consumed during Super Bowl week than any other week of the year.

SPINACH AND KALE TURNOVERS

MAKES 8 SERVINGS

In addition to being tasty, kale is a good source of lutein, benefiting eye health, and immunity-boosting vitamins A and C. Serve this as a snack, or enjoy two turnovers as a meatless entrée. They are great made ahead and brown-bagged; reheat in a microwave or toaster oven.

2   *teaspoons extra virgin olive oil*
1   *cup chopped onion*
1   *garlic clove, chopped*
1   *bunch kale, blanched, squeezed dry and finely chopped*
1   *(8-ounce) package sliced mushrooms (button, cremini, or a blend)*
¼   *teaspoon salt*
½   *teaspoon freshly ground black pepper*
¾   *cup (3 ounces) crumbled feta cheese*
1   *(11.3-ounce) can refrigerated dinner roll dough (such as Pillsbury or Whole Foods Brand) Extra olive oil for brushing*
Optional: 2½ tablespoons grated fresh Parmesan cheese

1. Preheat oven to 375°F.
2. Prepare a baking sheet by greasing very lightly with olive oil.
3. Heat olive oil in a large skillet over medium-high heat. Add onion; sauté 10 minutes or until tender and lightly browned. Add garlic; sauté 2 minutes.
4. Add kale and mushrooms; sauté 8 minutes or until kale is tender. Stir in salt and pepper.
5. Remove from heat; cool slightly. Stir in feta.
6. Separate dough into 8 pieces. Roll each dough piece into a 5-inch circle.
7. Spoon about ⅓ cup kale mixture on half of each circle, leaving a ½-inch border. Fold dough over kale mixture until edges almost meet. Bring bottom edge of dough over top edge; crimp edges of dough with fingers to form a rim.
8. Place turnovers on baking sheet. Lightly coat turnovers with olive oil; sprinkle each turnover with about 1 teaspoon optional Parmesan.
9. Bake at 375°F for 18 minutes or until golden brown. Let stand at least 5 minutes before serving; serve warm or at room temperature.

SQUASH-AND-KALE TOASTS

MAKES 8 SERVINGS

No one will be able to resist the kale when it's combined with sweet roasted squash. You can use any kale for this recipe, but I love the way Lacinto kale (also known as Tuscan or dinosaur kale) works here.

2   *small delicata squash (2 pounds)—peeled, halved lengthwise, seeded and sliced crosswise ½-inch thick; you can also use butternut or another winter squash*

½ cup extra-virgin olive oil, plus more for
    brushing
Salt, to taste
Pepper, to taste
Tabasco or other hot sauce, to taste
1 bunch kale, deribbed, coarsely chopped
4 garlic cloves, minced
1 teaspoon (squirt of) lemon juice
8 ½-inch-thick slices of toasted sourdough,
    multi-grain, peasant, or gluten-free bread
Optional: 4 ounces shaved Parmigiano-Reggiano
    cheese (1½ loose cups)

1. Preheat the oven to 350°F.
2. In a medium bowl, toss the squash with 2 tablespoons of the olive oil and season with salt and pepper.
3. Spread the squash on a baking sheet and roast for about 30 minutes, turning once, until tender and lightly browned.
4. In a large skillet over medium heat, add the remaining ¼ cup plus 2 tablespoons of olive oil. Add the kale, salt to taste, and hot sauce. Sauté until kale grows soft, about 8 minutes.
5. Add the garlic to the kale and continue to sauté until kale is tender, about 3 minutes longer. Adjust seasonings as desired.
6. Add the squash to the skillet, squirt with lemon juice, and toss gently to combine.
7. Spoon the squash-kale mixture on the toasts, top with the optional shaved cheese, and serve.

LEMON LOVE

Lemon juice is a favorite culinary ingredient thanks to the bright, sunny flavor it gives savory and sweet food. But did you know that lemon juice also has health benefits? It's a digestive aid, helps flush toxins from the body, and is a diuretic that helps the body release stores of trapped water.

PICKLED KALE—THE PERFECT CONDIMENT

Pickled kale is yummy, savory, and puckery— a great accompaniment to sandwiches, but it's also fantastic on an appetizer plate. Be warned: You will be asked for the recipe.

1 tablespoon sesame oil
1 bunch Tuscan or regular kale, stemmed,
    leaves torn
2 tablespoons fish sauce (such as nam pla
    or nuoc nam)
¼ cup unseasoned rice vinegar

1. Heat oil in a large saucepan. Add kale; sauté until wilted, about 5 minutes.
2. Stir in fish sauce, then rice vinegar.
3. Allow to sit for 15 minutes before servings, for flavors to meld.

DIPS

LEMON-RICOTTA KALE DIP

MAKES ABOUT 2 CUPS

Here's a quick and easy dip that's bound to win nutrient-packed kale a few new fans. Serve with vegetable dippers or whole-grain crackers.

1   *bunch green kale, deribbed and finely chopped*
1   *large shallot, minced*
1   *garlic clove, minced*
¼   *cup water*
¾   *cup part-skim ricotta cheese*
1   *teaspoon sugar or honey*
   Juice and zest of 1 lemon
   Salt and pepper, to taste
   A splash of Tabasco or other hot sauce

1. In a large saucepan over medium heat, combine kale, shallot, garlic, and water. Cover. Cook, stirring occasionally, until vegetables are very tender, about 12 minutes. Add more water if the vegetables begin drying out.

2. Transfer vegetables and any liquid in the pan to a food processor and let cool a few minutes.

3. Add ricotta, sugar, lemon juice and zest, salt, pepper, and hot sauce. Pulse until mixture is smooth. Transfer to a bowl and serve.

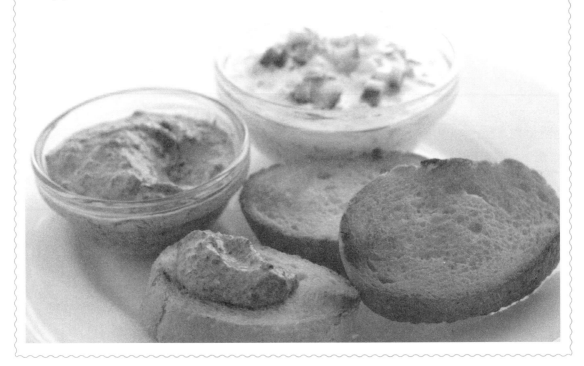

GARLICKY KALE AND SPINACH DIP

MAKES ABOUT 2 CUPS

This glorious dip is vegan, low-cal, and filled with antioxidants and powerful phytonutrients. Make this often—it's as delicious as it is virtuous.

1 cup cooked or steamed chopped kale, squeezed dry
1 cup cooked or steamed spinach, squeezed dry
2 medium garlic cloves, peeled
3 tablespoons toasted pine nuts
4 teaspoons balsamic vinegar
½ cup olive oil
Salt and pepper to taste

1. Add kale and spinach to the bowl of a food processor. Pulse until pureed.
2. Add garlic, pine nuts, and vinegar. Pulse to puree, slowly adding in the olive oil.
3. Scrape down the bowl, add salt and pepper, and pulse to blend.

GREEN SURPRISE DIP

MAKES 2½ CUPS

A delicious dip perfect for crudités, chips, or other dippers. It is also great as a sandwich spread or binder for chicken or tuna salad!

1 cup cooked or steamed kale, squeezed dry
1 cup plain yogurt (non-dairy yogurt is fine)
1 cup canned chickpeas, rinsed and drained
¼ cup mayonnaise
2 cloves garlic
½ onion, minced
1 tablespoon lemon juice or to taste
Salt to taste

1. Place all ingredients in a food processor or blender and puree until smooth.

CHOOSE YOUR PART

Almost all parts of some brassica species or other have been developed for food, including the root (rutabaga, turnips), stems (kohlrabi), leaves (cabbage, kale), flowers (cauliflower, broccoli, Brussels sprouts), and seeds (mustard seed, and oil-producing rapeseed).

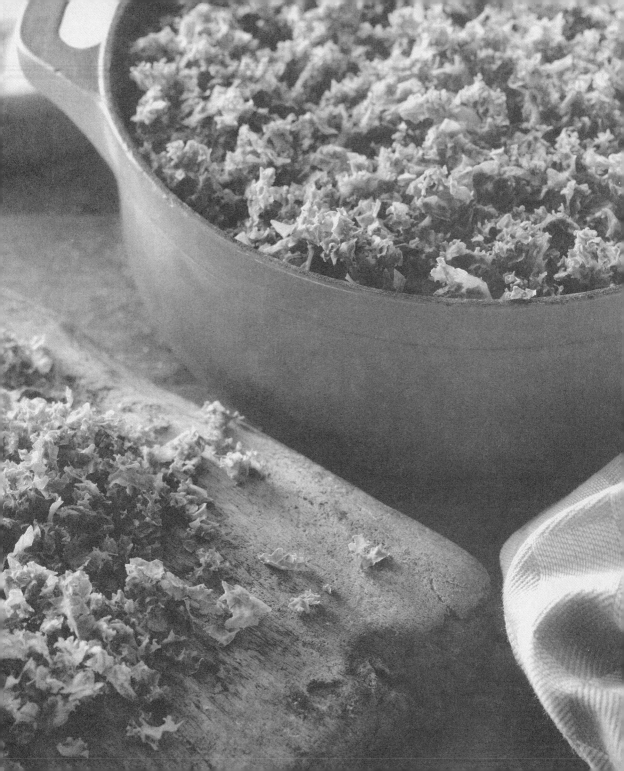

CHAPTER 7

KALE FOR DINNER

In many countries—including ours less than a century ago—the last meal of the day was light and nourishing and casual. A bowl of soup or a salad or a sandwich eaten a few hours before bedtime and you were ready to relax and unwind from a long day of farm or factory work.

Today we do things a bit differently—dinner is a big deal, and for most people, it's also the largest meal of the day. It's a time to gather with friends or family to create a shared experience. It's also much less casual than it used to be, meaning many people feel pressured to "create a meal," something yummy and spectacular (or at least a bit showy). The drawback to this fancier way of eating? Health considerations often fly out the window.

Fortunately, you can keep dinner the entertaining meal you enjoy and look out for your health simply by adding nutritious ingredients, such as kale, to your menu. Plus, when kale is for dinner, you can be sure that you and those you are feeding, are getting the best nutrition on the planet, including omega-3s, vitamins, minerals, fiber, plant protein, antioxidants, amino acids, and more.

ENTREES

CHICKEN KALE BRAISE
MAKES 4 SERVINGS

Braising is a moist, covered way of cooking vegetables and meats that creates a tender, succulent finish. Feel free to use different chicken parts or even remove the skin if you'd like. You can even swap the olive oil for coconut oil and add a ½ tablespoon or more of your favorite curry powder. Serve with your favorite grain.

3   *tablespoons extra virgin olive oil, divided*
4   *chicken leg quarters, skinned*
½   *teaspoon freshly ground black pepper*
¼   *teaspoon salt*
¼   *cup all-purpose flour*
5   *garlic cloves, minced*
2   *cups coarsely chopped kale*
1   *(14.5-ounce) can diced tomatoes, undrained (I like Muir Glen's Diced Tomato with Basil or Fire Roasted Tomatoes)*
1   *(14.5-ounce) can chicken broth*
1   *tablespoon red wine vinegar*

1. Preheat oven to 325°F.
2. In a shallow baking dish, mix together pepper, salt, and flour.
3. Dredge chicken in flour mixture, making sure chicken is completely covered.
4. Heat a Dutch oven pan over medium-high heat. Add 1 tablespoon oil. Place 2 leg quarters in pan, and cook for 1½ minutes on each side, just to brown. Remove from pan. Add another tablespoon of oil and remaining 2 chicken pieces, cooking each 1 to 1½ minutes on each side to brown. Set chicken aside.
5. Do not clean pan. Add another tablespoon of oil, then add garlic, cooking for a minute.
6. Add kale to the pan, cooking until just wilted, about 5 minutes.
7. Add tomatoes with their juice, and broth. Bring to a boil, stirring frequently
8. Remove pan from heat, add chicken, cover with lid, and place in oven.
9. Bake for about 65 to 75 minutes, until chicken loses its pinkness and juices run clear.
10. Stir in vinegar. Serve chicken over kale.

CHICKEN WITH KALE LENTIL PILAF

MAKES 4 SERVINGS

This healthy, nourishing dish is so comforting. It's also easy. It's great for a family meal. If you'd like to take it to a potluck or buffet, chop the chicken into a medium dice and stir into the grain-kale mixture.

ARSENIC AND WHAT ELSE IN OUR CHICKEN?

My first encounter with arsenic-tainted chicken came after one of my son's blood tests came back showing dangerously high levels of arsenic. The doctor quizzed us a bit on my son's habits and his favorite foods. When I said "chicken," the doctor said, "Aha! That's where the arsenic is coming from." It turns out that in the United States, arsenic is routinely been fed to poultry (and sometimes hogs) because it reduces infections and gives the flesh an appetizing shade of pinkness. If you want your poultry without toxic heavy metals, go organic.

VINAIGRETTE

1   to 2 teaspoons cumin powder
¼   cup sherry vinegar
1   garlic clove, minced
¼   cup extra-virgin olive oil
1   tablespoon finely chopped raisins
1   teaspoon whole grain mustard
1   teaspoon fresh lemon juice
    Salt to taste

PILAF AND CHICKEN

4   tablespoons extra virgin olive oil, divided
1½ pounds skinless, boneless chicken breast cutlets
    Salt to taste
1   tablespoon unsalted butter
1   garlic clove, minced
1   bunch kale, deribbed and finely chopped

2 cups cooked grain (quinoa, millet, brown rice, etc.)
1 cup cooked lentils

1. Add cumin, vinegar, garlic, oil, raisins, mustard, lemon juice, and salt to a blender. Whir to puree. Set aside.
2. Season chicken with salt.
3. Heat 2 tablespoons oil in a large heavy nonstick skillet over medium heat. Working in two batches and adding 1 tablespoon oil between batches, cook chicken in single layers until browned on both sides and just cooked through, 2 to 3 minutes per side. Transfer to a plate and cover loosely with foil to keep warm.
4. Remove pan from heat; add ¼ cup water. Stir, scraping up browned bits. Whisk in ¼ cup vinaigrette. Scrape sauce into a bowl.

5. Melt butter with 1 tablespoon oil in same skillet over medium-low heat. Add garlic and cook until just beginning to soften, about 1 minute.
6. Working in 3 batches and adding more oil as needed, add kale to skillet and toss until wilted, about 2 minutes. Transfer kale to a large bowl, season lightly with salt and cover with foil to keep warm.
7. Do not clean out pan. Instead, add grain and lentils to the same skillet, turn the heat to medium-high, and sauté for 2 minutes, or until warmed through.
8. Add rice-lentil mixture to kale, stir to combine.
9. To serve, spoon pilaf onto plates. Top with chicken. Drizzle dressing over chicken and pilaf.

CUMIN: DID YOU KNOW....?

- Cumin seed's scientific name is *Cuminum cyminum*.
- The seed is a rich source of iron, a mineral that plays many vital roles in the body.
- In many cultures, including the West Indies, India, Pakistan, and Mexico, cumin is used as a digestive aid. Recent research has indeed found that cumin stimulates the secretion of pancreatic enzymes, which help with digestion and nutrient assimilation.
- Cumin boasts anti-carcinogenic properties. In one study, cumin was shown to protect laboratory animals from developing stomach or liver tumors.
- High in antioxidants, cumin enhances the body's immune system function.

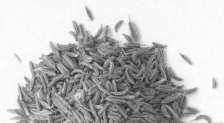

KALE MUSHROOM POLENTA

MAKES 6 SERVINGS

Polenta is another comfort food, this one from Italy. If you've never eaten polenta before, it's basically savory porridge, made nowadays with corn meal. Adding kale and mushroom makes this a meal. Note: There is quite a lot of dairy in this recipe. Feel free to use non-dairy (unsweetened) milk, butter, and cheese.

1¼ pounds cooked, steamed or blanched kale, deribbed, coarsely chopped
4   cups milk
3½ cups water
2   cups stone ground corn meal
½   teaspoon salt
¾   teaspoon ground black pepper
4   ounces pancetta (Italian bacon) or no-nitrite bacon, coarsely chopped
4   ounces mushrooms (such as button crimini, oyster, and stemmed shiitake), sliced
4   tablespoons extra-virgin olive oil, divided
1   garlic clove, minced
½   cup chicken broth
1   tablespoon chopped fresh thyme or parsley or basil
4   tablespoons unsalted butter
⅔   cup freshly grated Parmesan cheese

1. In a large, heavy saucepan over medium heat, bring milk, water, polenta, salt, and pepper to boil, whisking constantly. Once the mixture hits a rolling boil, reduce heat

MORE ON MUSHROOMS

- A mushroom is the fleshy, spore-bearing fruiting body of a fungus, typically produced above ground on soil or on its food source.
- Mushrooms are the only natural fresh vegetable or fruit that contains Vitamin D.
- There are about 300 species of edible mushrooms.
- One serving of mushrooms is equivalent to 5 white button mushrooms.
- One serving of mushrooms contains only 20 calories.
- Mushrooms boast high levels of antioxidants, making them a popular healing food in herbal medicine and other alternative nutrition therapies.
- Pennsylvania produces 65% of the mushrooms grown in the U.S.
- September is National Mushroom Month.
- The average American eats almost 4 pounds of mushrooms per year.
- White, or button, mushrooms are the most popular mushroom followed by criminis.
- Almost 90% of all consumers use mushrooms as an ingredient in recipes.

immediately to low and simmer until mixture is thickened, about 20 minutes, stirring occasionally (you may need to switch to a spoon). Remove from heat.

2. Meanwhile, in heavy large skillet over medium-high heat, cook pancetta until golden brown, about 3 minutes. Using slotted spoon, transfer pancetta to paper towels. Do not wipe out pan.

3. Add mushrooms and 2 tablespoons oil to drippings in skillet. Sauté until mushrooms are tender, about 5 minutes. Stir in kale and pancetta. Add garlic and broth; simmer for about 5 or 6 minutes.

4. Stir in thyme, salt, and pepper.

5. Whisk butter and Parmesan into polenta until smooth. Spoon polenta attractively on plates and top with kale mixture.

NONA'S PASTA

MAKES 6 SERVINGS

Though it has grandma in the name, my husband is the one who first made this for me, back in our early rock-n-roll days we ate a lot of lentils and other legumes, as well as pasta. He learned this dish from his Sicilian grandmother. I find it faster to use already-cooked lentils and blanched kale, but you can start from scratch.

2 cups (you can use up to 4 cups if desired) cooked lentils (make sure they are a bit firm; you don't want mushy lentils in this dish)
   Salt, to taste
   Pepper, to taste
6 tablespoons extra-virgin olive oil
1 large onion, finely chopped
1 or 2 garlic cloves, minced
1 bunch kale, deribbed, blanched, squeezed dry and coarsely chopped.
½ cup chicken broth (or salted water)
1 pound dried elbow or ditalini or other short tubular pasta, cooked to al dente
Optional: Parmegiano-Reggiano cheese to grate over the top

1. In a large heavy skillet over medium-high heat, warm ¼ cup oil until hot but not smoking. Sauté onion and garlic with pepper and salt, stirring, for about 1 minute. Reduce heat to low and cook, covered, stirring occasionally, until onions are soft and golden (stir more frequently toward end of cooking), about 20 minutes. Remove lid and increase heat to moderate, then cook, stirring frequently, until onion is golden brown, 5 to 10 minutes more.

2. Add all remaining ingredients, stir, and increase heat to high. Cover pan and allow to cook for about 1 minute.

3. Adjust seasoning with salt and pepper before serving.

KALE-PORK GRATIN

MAKES 4 SERVINGS

I adore gratins! They are toasty, tasty, easy, and versatile. And, every single time I make one, everyone smiles, there is no complaining, and everyone (my four-year-old included) finishes their dinner. (Even if it contains kale.)

5   *to 6 cups cooked, steamed or blanched kale, squeezed dry, deribbed, and finely chopped*
    Salt to taste
3   *tablespoons extra-virgin olive oil*
¼   *pound pancetta, ham, bacon, chopped into ½-inch pieces*
1   *cup cream*
2   *to 3 cloves garlic, minced*
    Black pepper to taste
½   *cup breadcrumbs (you can use gluten-free bread)*
½   *cup grated Parmigiano-Reggiano or Pecorino Romano*

1. Preheat the broiler, adjusting the oven rack on the second shelf down from the heat source.
2. In a large skillet over medium-high heat, add 1 tablespoon of olive oil and pancetta. Cook until pancetta is crisp and add cream and garlic.
3. Crisp the pancetta and add the cream and garlic. Season salt and pepper.
4. Continue cooking until mixture has reduced to about ½ to ⅔ cups (you can eyeball this), about 7 to 9 minutes.
5. Add kale to cream and stir to coat evenly.
6. Transfer mixture to a shallow casserole dish.

7. In a medium bowl, mix together breadcrumbs, remaining 2 tablespoons of extra-virgin olive oil, salt, pepper, and cheese. Sprinkle over kale mixture in the casserole dish.
8. Place the casserole on the second shelf under broiler and cook until breadcrumbs are brown, about 5 minutes.

GRATIN CHRONICLES

Quick! What do you think of when I say the word "gratin"? Something with a bubbly, cheesy, crumbly topping? If so, you're right on. Gratin is the French term for any food that is topped with a browned crust, often using breadcrumbs, grated cheese, egg, and/or butter. French in origin, the term comes from the word grater, which means "to scrape" or "grate." Original gratins were prepared in a shallow dish and topped with some kind of crumbly mixture, before being browned in the oven or under a broiler.

PORK MADE HEALTHY

Pork has a reputation for being a fatty, unhealthy meat. And while bacon, cracklins, and high-fat sausages aren't the most health-supportive choices, pork has a lot of redeeming features. Choose a lean pork cut such as tenderloin and you've got a meal that is lower in fat than beef, high in zinc and protein, and rich in thiamin, a B-vitamin that helps your body create and use energy.

FAST FETTUCCINE WITH KALE AND SAUSAGE

MAKES 4 SERVINGS

My kids and my hubby adore Italian sausage, so they'll eat pretty much anything if it has sausage in it. This is a fun way to combine sausage and kale. If you're gluten-free (like two of my sons), use a gluten-free pasta here. (My favorite is Tinkyada brand.)

3   tablespoons olive oil
1   pound hot turkey or pork sausage, casings discarded and sausage crumbled
½   lb kale, deribbed, blanched, squeezed dry and coarsely chopped
    Salt
½   pound dry fettuccine pasta
⅔   cup chicken broth
¼   to ½ cup finely grated Pecorino Romano

1. Heat oil in a 12-inch heavy skillet over moderately high heat until hot but not smoking. Cook sausage until browned, 5 to 7 minutes, breaking up any lumps with a spoon.

2. Meanwhile, fill large pot with salted water and bring to a boil. Cook pasta in boiling water, uncovered, until al dente. Reserve 1 cup pasta-cooking water, then drain pasta in a colander. (If using gluten-free pasta, follow instructions on the bag.)

3. While the pasta cooks, add blanched kale to sausage in skillet and sauté, stirring frequently, until kale is just tender, about 5 minutes.

4. Add broth, stirring and scraping up any brown bits from bottom of skillet, then add pasta and ½ cup reserved cooking water to skillet, tossing until combined. Stir in cheese and thin with additional cooking water if desired.

ONE-POT GREEN PENNE

MAKES 6 SERVINGS

Once upon a time, when my husband and I were vegan, we ate a lot of pasta. Then I began studying nutrition and realized two things: I don't digest wheat and hubby needs occasional animal protein to be his healthiest. The result? We cut way back on pasta. That said, I still make this yummy recipe today, but to accommodate everyone in my household, I often use gluten-free pasta.

¼ cup chopped fresh basil or Italian parsley (or a blend)
Squirt of lemon juice
1 teaspoon finely grated lemon peel
2 garlic cloves, minced
1 bunch kale, deribbed and coarsely chopped
1 pound penne (you can use gluten-free if you'd like)
5 tablespoons extra-virgin olive oil, divided
½ cup coarsely chopped pitted Kalamata olives
½ cup crumbled feta cheese (about 3 ounces)
Salt and pepper to taste

OLIVE OIL: DID YOU KNOW....?

- The olive tree is native to the Mediterranean.
- Spain is the world's largest overall producer of olive oil. Italy is second.
- In Homer's *Odyssey*, the Phoenician princess Nausicaa carries a golden flask filled with olive oil. She and her maids anoint themselves with the oil after bathing in the river. In Ancient Greece and other Mediterranean countries, men and women applied olive oil to their skin and hair after bathing as a moisturizer and to protect their hair and skin from the elements.
- In Greece, women created eye shadow by mixing ground charcoal with olive oil.
- In Homer's *Iliad*, Aphrodite anoints the dead body of Hector with rose-scented olive oil. This was common in Ancient Greece, where bodies were often treated with olive oil to mask the smell of decomposition.
- Olive oil played an important role in early athletic events. Before working out or competing, Greek athletes rubbed their naked bodies with olive oil to protect themselves from the sun and to help regulate body temperature. Once their competition was over, the athletes would use a tool called a "strigil" and scrape away the oil, sweat, and dirt from their skin.
- In Rome, pregnant women applied olive oil to their skin to prevent stretch marks. Women today still do this.
- In the Bible, King Solomon uses olive oil to buy wood to build his temple.
- Christopher Columbus introduced olive oil to South and Central America in 1492.
- Olive trees were taken north from Mexico into California in the 1700s.
- Olive oil didn't become commonplace in the United States until the late 1800s and early 1900s, when Greek, Italian, and Spanish immigrants began importing it from their homelands.
- Italy exports more olive oil to the United States than to anywhere else.

1. Mix basil, lemon juice, lemon peel, and garlic in small bowl; set aside.

2. Bring large pot of salted water to boil. Add kale and cook just until tender, about 6 or 7 minutes. Using skimmer or slotted spoon, transfer greens to colander to drain.

3. Return water to boil. Add pasta and cook just until tender but still firm to bite, stirring occasionally. Drain, reserving ¾ cup pasta cooking liquid.

4. Return pasta to pot; add greens and 3 tablespoons oil and toss. Stir in olives, feta, and enough reserved pasta cooking liquid by ¼ cupfuls to moisten.

5. Stir herb-lemon mixture and remaining olive oil into the pasta and greens. Season with salt and pepper.

PORK CHOPS WITH KALE CHIP GREMOLATA

MAKES 4 SERVINGS

I first tasted gremolata in a cooking class, where I was a kitchen assistant. The instructor had given me and the other assistant some leftover cooked potatoes with the remaining tablespoons of the gremolata she had just made. I had never tasted anything so bright and sunny! What's different in this version is instead of parsley, you are using kale. The results are delicious! Use any extras to dress up sandwiches, salads, eggs, and poultry.

½ small bunch kale, deribbed
¾ cup olive oil
    Salt, to taste
    Pepper, to taste
½ cup walnut pieces
4 center-cut bone-in pork chops, about ¾-inch thick (2 pounds total)
¼ teaspoon dried rosemary, crushed with your fingers
1 small clove garlic, quartered
    Pinch crushed red pepper flakes
2 tablespoons fresh lemon juice
Optional: 1 teaspoon lemon zest
    Baked potato or soft polenta, for serving

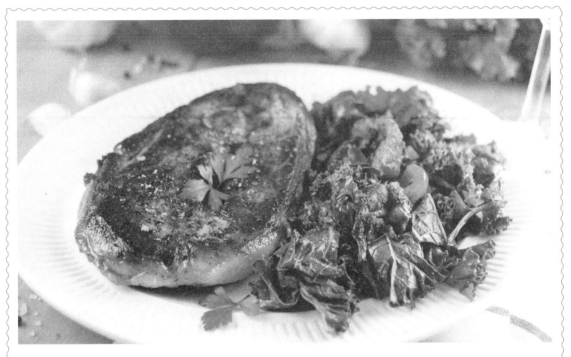

1. Preheat the broiler.

2. In a large bowl, gently toss the kale leaves with two tablespoons of olive oil and ¼ teaspoon salt. Spread them in an even layer on a baking sheet

3. Place the baking sheet under the broiler, stirring greens once or twice until they are bright in color with charred edges, about 4 or 5 minutes.

4. Toss walnuts onto the baking sheet with the kale leaves and broil for another minute or two, until the walnuts are toasty but not burned. Set kale and walnuts aside to cool.

5. Sprinkle both sides of the chops with ½ teaspoon salt, ¼ teaspoon pepper, and the rosemary.

6. In a large skillet over medium heat, add 2 tablespoons of the olive oil. Add the pork chops and cook, turning once, until the meat is done. Do not over-cook. Transfer to a plate to rest for 5 minutes.

7. While the chops are cooking, add the garlic and the cooled kale and walnuts to the bowl of a food processor and pulse until chopped. Add the pepper flakes, lemon juice, optional lemon zest, ¼ teaspoon salt, and the remaining ½ cup olive oil and continue to process to make a slightly chunky pesto. Adjust the consistency as desired with up to ¼ cup water. Season to taste with salt and pepper.

8. Top each pork chop with about 2 tablespoons of the gremolata.

SPICY CHICKEN KALE STIR-FRY

MAKES 4 SERVINGS

Every cook (and non-cook) needs a good stir-fry recipe. This one is mine. I love the nutty flavor, as do my kids. I also love the healthy ingredients. Leftovers are good packed up and eaten for lunch the next day. Serve this over brown rice, quinoa, or millet.

2   tablespoons tamari (or other soy sauce)
1   teaspoon minced fresh ginger
1   clove garlic, minced
2   tablespoons dry sherry
3   teaspoons toasted sesame oil
2   teaspoons golden brown sugar
1¼ pounds skinless boneless chicken breast
      halves, cut crosswise into thin strips,
      then chopped into chunks
3   tablespoons virgin coconut oil divided
4   scallions, sliced thinly, including the light
      green sections
1   small jalapeno chili, seeds and veins removed,
      then finely chopped
1   bunch kale, deribbed, and coarsely chopped
Optional: Two tablespoons chopped cilantro
      leaves
Optional: ¼ cup chopped roasted salted peanuts,
      cashews, almonds, or walnuts

1. In a medium bowl, whisk tablespoon tamari, ginger, garlic, sherry, sesame oil, and sugar in medium bowl. Pour half of this liquid into a measuring cup or other container to reserve. Add chicken to the bowl and allow to marinade for 20 to 30 minutes.

2. Heat 2 tablespoons oil in large nonstick skillet over high heat. Add scallion and jalapeno, stirring for 30 seconds.

3. Add chicken to the skillet and stir-fry just until cooked through, about 3 minutes. Transfer chicken mixture to bowl and set aside.

4. Add 1 tablespoon oil to same skillet; heat over high heat. Add greens by large handfuls; stir just until beginning to wilt before adding more. Sauté just until tender, about 6 to 8 minutes.

5. Return chicken to skillet. Add reserved soy sauce mixture; stir until heated through, about one minute. Season with salt and pepper.

6. Transfer to serving bowl; sprinkle with optional cilantro and nuts.

SESAME: THE BACTERIA BUSTER

Sesame oil is known for both its antioxidant and antibacterial activity, which makes it a popular protective skin treatment and dietary supplement. But did you know that sesame oil is also a popular herbal cure for gingivitis and cavities? Swish 2 or more tablespoons of cold-pressed sesame oil around in the mouth for 2 or more minutes. Gargle if desired.

SIDE DISHES

CREAMED KALE

MAKES 6 SERVINGS

You're probably familiar with the original spinach version of this dish. For some people (I know you're not one of them!), creamed spinach is the only green veggie they'll eat. Do you have anyone like that in your life? If so, let me help you shake up their food world with Creamed Kale. Note: This is a pretty dairy-intensive dish, so you'll want to make this a "once in awhile" dish. You can play around with non-dairy alternatives if you'd like, but I haven't had a lot of luck with them. Just being honest.

3   *pounds kale, deribbed, blanched, squeezed dry and coarsely chopped*
3½ *cups whole milk, or more if needed*
3   *tablespoons unsalted butter, plus more for the baking dish*
1   *medium Spanish onion, finely diced*
1   *small shallot, finely diced*
3   *cloves garlic, finely chopped*
3   *tablespoons all-purpose flour*
Optional: ⅛ teaspoon freshly grated nutmeg
      Salt, to taste
      Pepper, to taste

1. Preheat the oven to 350°F.
2. Butter a 10-inch square baking dish.
3. Pour the milk into a medium saucepan and bring to a simmer over low heat.
4. Melt the butter in a medium saucepan over medium-high heat. Add the onion and shallot and cook until soft, about 5 minutes. Add the garlic and cook for 30 seconds.
5. Whisk in the flour and cook until smooth and light blonde in color, about 1 minute.
6. Slowly whisk in the warm milk, raise the heat to high, and cook, whisking constantly, until thickened and the flour taste has cooked out, about 5 minutes. If the mixture becomes too thick, add a little more milk.
7. Strain the sauce over the kale. Add the optional nutmeg, season with salt and pepper, and mix gently to combine. Scrape the mixture into the baking dish and bake in the oven until light golden brown on top and just warmed through, about 15 minutes.

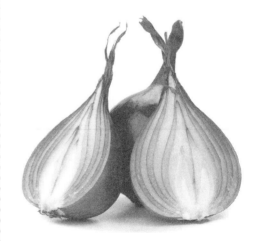

GREEN POLENTA

MAKES 6 SERVINGS

Here's another green recipe. Literally. Hey if you're going to eat healthfully, why not have a little fun? Fortunately, this easy recipe is also delicious. Your kids will love it. Try it with poultry, meats, or vegetable ragouts.

2   *tablespoons extra virgin olive oil*
½   *onion, diced*
3   *cloves garlic, minced*
1   *bunch kale, deribbed and coarsely chopped*
    Salt, to taste
    Pepper, to taste
5   *cups chicken broth*
2½ *cups heavy cream*
1½ *cups stone-ground corn meal*
6   *tablespoons butter*
4   *tablespoons grated Parmesan*

1. In a large sauté pan, heat the olive oil over medium heat. Add the onions and sauté until translucent, about 3 minutes.
2. Add the garlic and kale, season with salt and pepper to taste, and cook until wilted. Set aside to cool.
3. In another large pot, bring 5 cups of broth and 2 cups heavy cream to a boil over medium heat. Whisk in the corn meal and stir constantly until the polenta is creamy, about 20 minutes. If the mixture becomes too thick, add a little water.
4. When the kale mixture has cooled, add it to the bowl of a food processor. Process until mixture is a smooth, velvety, green puree. If the mixture seems thick and chunky, add a bit of water or broth and process again.
5. Stir butter into the cooked polenta and season with salt and pepper, to taste. Fold in the kale and the Parmesan.

THE HISTORY OF POLENTA

Once upon a time, polenta—known in the days of ancient Rome as pulmentum—was a humble, everyday grain mush (think porridge) eaten by everyone and made from any starchy ingredient, including farro, chestnut flour, millet, spelt, or ground chickpeas. With the introduction of corn in the 16th century, corn became the de rigueur ingredient for proper polenta.

FRIED PORK RICE WITH KALE

MAKES 1 TO 2 SERVINGS

Do you have your local Chinese food takeout place on speed dial? It's time to take your culinary power back and learn how to make fried rice yourself. It's easy. I promise. And fun! Use cold, leftover rice for this. Freshly-cooked rice will not give you the right results. If you don't have pork tenderloin, use a leftover pork chop or chicken meat. Or leave out the animal protein altogether.

2   tablespoons sesame oil
2   garlic cloves, minced
1   tablespoon finely minced fresh ginger
1   small onion, halved lengthwise and thinly
     sliced crosswise
1   carrot, cut into ⅛-inch-thick matchsticks
¾   cup steamed or cooked kale, squeezed dry
     and finely chopped
½   cup red bell pepper, cut into thin, short strips
1½ cups chilled cooked rice such as short grain
     brown rice
½   to ¾ cup roast pork tenderloin, cut crosswise
     into ⅓-inch-thick slices and slices cut into
     ⅓-inch-wide strips
1   tablespoon rice wine vinegar
1   tablespoon tamari or other soy sauce
1   teaspoon brown sugar or honey
2   scallions, thinly sliced
Optional: 1 teaspoon minced fresh jalapeno or
     Serrano chili
Optional: 2 tablespoons chopped fresh cilantro
Optional: 1 large egg, lightly beaten (optional)

1. Heat oil in a wok or a deep 12-inch heavy nonstick skillet over moderately high heat until hot but not smoking. Add garlic and ginger and stir-fry until golden, about 1 minute.

2. Add onion and stir-fry until lightly browned, about 2 minutes.

3. Add carrot, kale, and red pepper and stir-fry 2 minutes.

4. Add rice and pork and stir-fry 1 minute.

5. In a small bowl, whisk together rice vinegar, tamari, honey, and chili until honey is dissolved.

6. Add soy mixture to wok, then add scallions and 1 tablespoon optional cilantro and stir-fry for one minute.

7. Add optional beaten egg and stir-fry until egg is set, about 1 minute.

8. Serve sprinkled with remaining tablespoon cilantro.

SODIUM AND SOY SAUCE

Soy sauce is used as a salty flavoring and condiment in several Asian countries. It is delicious stuff! But keep in mind that soy sauce is high in sodium. A single tablespoon of the stuff can contain up to 1,000 mg of sodium. Current dietary guidelines recommend that you get no more than 2,300 mg a day, with a healthier daily sodium intake being 1,500 mg or less. (Just to put all this sodium talk in context: Most American adults ingest 3,266 mg per day in convenience food—that's not even counting table salt that's added to food.)

GREEN POTATO PUREE

MAKES 8 SERVINGS

This is bright green. Yes it is. So bright, that people may think it is creamed spinach. It's actually better (in my opinion): A velvety, hearty puree that pairs beautifully with poultry and red meat, and makes a fun bed to sit fish atop. Thin leftovers with a bit of chicken broth for a lovely soup.

2   *pounds kale, deribbed, coarsely chopped*
1½ *pounds large boiling potatoes, peeled and*
       cut into half-inch cubes
2   *cups heavy cream*
       Salt, to taste
       Pepper, to taste

1. Fill a large pot with salted water and place, uncovered over a high flame. When the water begins to boil, add kale, cooking it until tender, about 7 minutes.

KALE TRIVIA

In nineteenth century Scotland "kail" was used as a generic term for "dinner" and all kitchens featured a "kail-pot" for cooking.

2. Quickly drain kale and run cold water over the greens to stop the cooking process. Set wet, cooled greens aside.

3. While kale cooks, place a heavy medium saucepan over medium heat, adding potatoes, cream, salt, and pepper. Simmer, covered, stirring occasionally, until tender, 15 to 20 minutes.

4. Add the kale to the bowl of a food processor, processing until absolutely smooth.

5. Add potatoes, and pulse until smooth.

6. Serve immediately, or transfer to a large heavy saucepan and heat through before serving.

THE POTATO EATERS: DID YOU KNOW...?

- The average American eats 137.9 pounds of potatoes each year.
- 50.7 pounds of the potatoes consumed each year are fresh.
- 55.3 pounds of the potatoes consumed each year are frozen potato products, such as French fries, hash browns, etc.
- 16.9 pounds of the potatoes consumed each year are as potato chips.
- 13 pounds of the potatoes consumed each year are dehydrated potato products, such as boxed potato flakes, au gratin mixes, and so on.
- 2 pounds of the potatoes consumed each year are canned potatoes, found in soup and other canned products.

HEARTY WINTER SALAD

MAKES 4 SERVINGS

This is truly a cold-weather salad. Heavy, hearty, rib-sticking—it's also rich in nutrients and tastes wonderful.

2 *pounds Yukon Gold potatoes, cut into 1-inch pieces*
⅓ *cup extra virgin olive oil*
4 *garlic cloves (3 thinly sliced and 1 left whole)*
¼ *cup well-stirred tahini*
2 *tablespoons water*
3 *tablespoons fresh lemon juice*
1 *bunch kale, deribbed and leaves cut in a chiffonade*
 Salt, to taste
 Pepper, to taste

1. Preheat oven to 450°F with a rack in upper third.
2. In a large bowl, mix potatoes with oil and ½ teaspoon each of salt and pepper. Tossing until potatoes are coated. Transfer potatoes to a baking pan, spreading them in an even layer. Place in oven and roast, for about 12 minutes, stirring once.
3. Stir in sliced garlic and roast 12 minutes more.
4. In the bowl of a food processor purée tahini, water, lemon juice, fourth (whole) garlic clove, and ½ teaspoon salt in a blender until smooth, about 1 minute. Add a bit of water if sauce is too thick.
5. Toss kale with hot potatoes and any garlic and oil remaining in pan, then toss with tahini sauce and salt and pepper to taste.

KALE CASSEROLE

MAKES 6 SERVINGS

I was raised on casseroles. They were at every church event I ever attended, every family reunion, and every single dinner I ever ate at home. (My mother, who didn't know how to cook, would open a can of condensed cream of mushroom soup and dump it into a Pyrex casserole dish, then add a 1 cup of canned or frozen veggies, 1 cup of leftover meat (or a can of tuna), 1 cup of leftover Minute Rice or noodles, then top the thing with a handful of saltine crackers she'd put in a plastic bag and crushed with the bottom of a drinking glass.) I was well into adulthood before I could even get near another casserole, but with a bit of perspective, I realize that casseroles are good things: Easy, economical, nourishing, and fast. This one, which contains no cream of mushroom soup, is also vegetarian and dressy enough for a holiday table.

FOR VEGETABLES

2 *tablespoons olive oil*
2 *medium onions, halved lengthwise and thinly sliced lengthwise*
1 *pound cabbage, cored and cut crosswise into ⅓-inch-thick slices (4 cups)*
1 *pound kale, stems and center ribs removed and leaves coarsely chopped (12 cups)*
½ *pound carrots, cut into ¼-inch-thick matchsticks*
½ *cup water*
2 *tablespoons soy sauce*
½ *teaspoon salt*

FOR TOPPING

1½ *cups fine fresh or dried bread crumbs, preferably whole wheat*
7 *ounces firm tofu*
1 *ounce finely grated Parmigiano-Reggiano (½ cup)*
⅓ *cup olive oil*
2 *teaspoons dried basil, crumbled*

1½ *teaspoons dried oregano, crumbled*
1 *teaspoon paprika*
1 *garlic clove, chopped*
¼ *teaspoon salt*

1. Put oven rack in middle position and preheat oven to 350°F.

2. Heat oil in a deep 12- to 14-inch heavy skillet over moderately high heat until hot but not smoking, then sauté onion, stirring occasionally, until softened and beginning to brown, about 5 minutes. Reduce heat to moderate and add cabbage, kale, carrots, water, soy sauce, and salt. (Skillet will be full, but volume will reduce as vegetables steam.) Cook, covered, stirring occasionally, until vegetables are just tender, 10 to 15 minutes. Transfer to a 13- by 9-inch glass baking dish.

3. Make topping: Pulse all topping ingredients together in a food processor until combined well. Alternatively, mash ingredients together in a large bowl with a potato masher. Sprinkle tofu mixture over vegetables in baking dish and bake, uncovered, until topping is golden brown and vegetables are heated through, 15 to 20 minutes.

THE STORY BEHIND THE WORD

In the United States, the word "casserole" is synonymous with church suppers, potlucks, and starchy, feed-lots-of-people dishes. The actual word, casserole, however, comes not from a food, but from a cooking vessel. Casserole is from the French word for "saucepan," a large, deep dish used both in the oven and as a serving vessel.

KALE MEAT PIES

MAKES 8 SERVINGS

I like meat pies. I don't care if they are from Jamaica, Australia, England or wherever. This tasty spin features our favorite green veggie, kale!

2½ cups all-purpose flour (spooned and leveled), plus more for rolling
1   cup (2 sticks) unsalted butter, cut into small pieces
1½ teaspoons fine salt
½   cup ice water
1   tablespoon extra-virgin olive oil
10 ounces (about 1½ links) sweet Italian sausage, casings removed
1   medium onion, diced medium
1   tart apple, such as Granny Smith, peeled and diced medium
1   bunch kale (¾ pound), tough stems and ribs removed, leaves coarsely chopped
¼   cup golden raisins
    Coarse salt and ground pepper
    Heavy cream, for brushing

1. In a food processor, pulse flour, butter, and salt until mixture resembles coarse meal, with a few pea-size pieces of butter remaining. With machine running, sprinkle with ¼ cup ice water; pulse just until dough holds together when squeezed (if necessary, add up to ¼ cup more water, 1 tablespoon at a time); do not overmix. Form dough into a disk, wrap tightly in plastic, and refrigerate 30 minutes (or up to overnight).

2. Meanwhile, in a large skillet, heat oil over medium-high. Add sausage and cook, breaking up meat with a wooden spoon, until browned, about 5 minutes.

3. Add onion and cook until translucent, about 6 minutes. Add apple, kale, and raisins and cook until kale is almost tender, about 5 minutes. Remove from heat; season with salt and pepper.

4. Preheat oven to 400°F. Line two baking sheets with parchment paper. On a lightly floured surface, roll out dough to an ⅛-inch thickness. With a large round cookie cutter or small bowl, cut out eight 6- to 7-inch rounds (reroll scraps if necessary).

5. Place ½ cup kale mixture in center of each round and fold over filling to form half-moons. With a fork, press edges firmly to seal. Place pies on baking sheets and brush with cream.

6. Cut a small vent in each pie and bake until golden brown and crisp, 25 to 30 minutes, rotating sheets halfway through. Let cool slightly on a wire rack. Serve warm or at room temperature.

KALE RICE

MAKES 2 SERVINGS

This is easy, fast, and yummy—the perfect side dish for serving alongside any type of animal protein, or veggie ragout, stew or bean dish. Everyone needs to know how to make this!

1   cup water or chicken broth
    Salt, to taste
    Pepper, to taste
½   cup long-grain brown rice (use basmati rice
    if you'd like)
2   small garlic cloves, minced
1   tablespoon olive oil
1   (14-ounce) can diced tomatoes, liquid reserved
    for another use
2   cups kale, deribbed, chopped finely

1. In a small heavy saucepan bring 1 cup water to a boil. Add the rice and salt to taste, then immediately cover the pot and turn the flame to low.

2. Cook the rice over low heat for 25 minutes, or until the liquid is absorbed and the rice is tender.

3. In a heavy skillet cook the garlic in the oil over moderately low heat, stirring, until it is soft.

4. Add the tomatoes and the kale to the skillet and cook the mixture, stirring occasionally, for 5 minutes, or until the kale is tender.

5. Dump the finished rice into a large bowl, fluff with fork, and add the kale mixture. Add salt and pepper, to taste. Mix gently until ingredients are combined.

RICE: DID YOU KNOW... ?

- Rice is the main dietary staple for more than half of the world's population.
- Rice has been cultivated for over 5,000 years.
- Arkansas is the largest producer of rice in the U.S. accounting for about 46% of U.S. rice production. California is the second largest rice producing state, growing about 17.7% of the U.S. rice crop on more than 500,000 acres.
- The U.S. exports about half of its rice crop, mostly to Mexico, Central America, Northeast Asia, the Caribbean, and the Middle East.
- September is National Rice Month.
- The first rice grown in the United States most likely came from Madagascar. It was planted in the Carolinas in the late 1680s.
- September is National Rice Month.
- It takes between 2,000 to 5,000 tons of water to produce a ton of rice.
- The major rice-producing states are Arkansas, California, Louisiana, Texas, Mississippi, and Missouri. Almost half of the U.S. rice crop is exported to over 100 countries.
- Rice is grown on every continent except Antarctica.
- Rice, millet, and sorghum are thought to be the first crops ever cultivated.
- Americans eat a little more than 24 pounds of rice per person each year. Asians eat as much as 300 pounds per person each year, while in the United Arab Emirates it is about 450 pounds, and in France about 10 pounds.

POTATO KALE CAKES

MAKES 12 SERVINGS

Unlike latkes, which are made with grated potatoes, these use mashed potatoes (yes, you can use leftovers!). The result is super elegant, super delicious, and pretty easy, too.

OPTIONAL SAUCE

½ cup mayonnaise
1 tablespoon extra-virgin olive oil
2 garlic cloves, minced
1 tablespoon tomato paste
⅛ teaspoon chipotle powder (use more if you can take the heat)
Salt, to taste
Pepper, to taste

POTATO CAKE

1½ pounds russet potatoes, peeled, cut into 1-inch cubes
¼ cup whole milk
2 tablespoons (¼ stick) unsalted butter
Salt, to taste
3½ tablespoons extra-virgin olive oil, divided
1 cup onion, minced
1 large garlic clove, minced
½ pound kale, deribbed, coarsely chopped
Optional: ½ teaspoon lemon zest

SAUCE DIRECTIONS

1. Whisk all ingredients in medium bowl. Can be made 1 day ahead. Cover and chill.

POTATO CAKE DIRECTIONS

1. Cook potatoes in large saucepan of boiling salted water until tender, about 25 minutes. Drain; return potatoes to same saucepan.

2. Add milk and butter. Mash potatoes until smooth. Season with ½ teaspoon coarse salt and ½ teaspoon pepper.

3. Transfer 3 cups mashed potatoes to large bowl and cool (reserve remaining potatoes for another use).

4. Heat 1½ tablespoons oil in large deep skillet over medium heat. Add onion and garlic. Sauté until onion softens, about 5 minutes.

5. Increase heat to medium-high. Add kale and cook until kale softens, about 7 minutes.

6. Add kale mixture, ½ teaspoon salt, and ½ teaspoon pepper to potatoes and thoroughly combine. Allow to sit for 45 minutes or more until mixture is thoroughly cool.

7. When the potato-kale mixture is cool, shape it by patting ¼-cup portions into patties about ½-inch thick. Keep shaping until all potato-kale mixture has been formed into patties.

8. Heat 2 tablespoons oil in large nonstick skillet over medium-high heat. Add patties and cook, without moving (you want a crust to form!), until they are brown and crispy on bottom, about 4 minutes.

9. Carefully turn cakes over. Cook until brown on bottom, about 3 minutes more. Transfer to plates. Top each cake with dollop of optional sauce, salsa, or other condiment.

THE POTATO: AMERICA'S FAVORITE VEGGIE

- The first potatoes arrived in North America in 1621 as a gift to Francis Wyatt, the Governor of Virginia at Jamestown. The tubers were sent via ship by Captain Nathaniel Butler, then governer of Bermuda.
- Though potatoes had been brought to the early American colonies by European explorers who'd brought the vegetable north from South America, they were believed to be poisonous. And were thus, avoided.
- Potatoes did not become popular until Benjamin Franklin fell in love with them while ambassador to France, then returned to the States to retire, bringing his love of potatoes with him.
- French fries were introduced to Americans when President Thomas Jefferson served them at the White House.

POTLIKER KALE

MAKES 2 SERVINGS

These are Southern-style greens, inspired by those long-simmered greens that are revered in the U.S. south. These have a decidedly shorter cooking time and a fresher taste, but use the same porky, puckery vinegar flavoring. And yes, of course you can omit the bacon—use a couple tablespoons of butter or your favorite oil, instead, and know that you'll have a completely different recipe.

1   *large bunch of kale, deribbed and chopped coarsely*
2   *bacon slices, chopped*
    Salt, to taste
    Pepper, to taste
2   *teaspoons cider vinegar, or to taste*

1. In a large heavy saucepan of boiling salted water boil kale for 5 minutes and drain well in colander.

2. In large skillet, cook bacon over moderate heat, stirring, until crisp.

3. Add kale to bacon and sauté over moderately high heat, stirring, until heated through.

4. Toss kale with vinegar and season with salt and pepper.

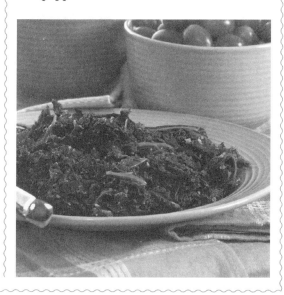

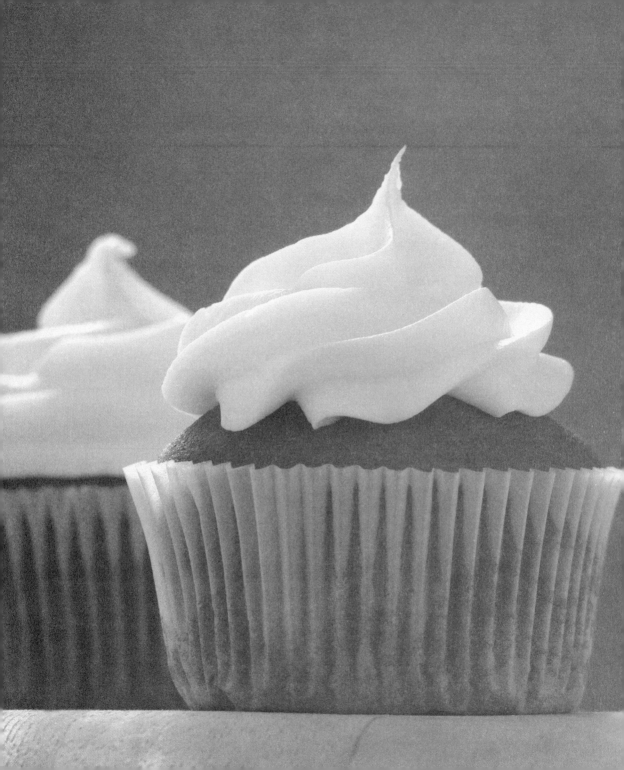

CHAPTER 8

DESSERTS & OTHER SWEETS

One of the wonderful benefits of eating lots of kale is improved hearing (it's the omega-3 fatty acids, magnesium, and vitamins A, C, and E—all of which have been shown to protect and improve hearing). In fact, my own hearing has become so good that I can hear you right now, as you read this chapter: "Kale in desserts?" you ask, incredulously. "That's just wrong!"

Perhaps, but it's also super healthy, super easy, and (yes!) super tasty! Sneaking a bit of kale into a sweet is an easy way to increase its nutrient profile and deliver a dose of nourishing kale to a picky kid (or adult); it's also terrific for gardeners who would feel terrible wasting even a leaf of their precious kale crop.

So go ahead and call me crazy, but do me a favor and try one of the recipes in this chapter. I have a feeling they'll make a "kale dessert convert" out of you. Just one bit of advice before you start: Baked goods should be allowed to completely cool to room temperature before serving. If they are the least bit warm, you will taste the kale.

BLUEBERRY KALE POPS

MAKES 4 TO 6 SERVINGS

Popsicles are a great place to slip in kale. The trick, however, is accompanying kale with dark, bold-tasting fruit. No kid wants a popsicle that tastes like frozen greens! That's why this fruity, refreshing recipe uses blueberries, kale, and grape juice, but feel free to experiment. The combinations are—quite literally—endless.

THE BEGINNING OF THE POPSICLE

- The first popsicle was invented in 1905 by an 11-year-old boy named Frank Epperson, who called his invention the Epsicle Ice Pop.
- Epperson invented the treat after leaving a cup of soda with a straw outdoors during the winter. It froze—and Epperson had himself a frozen treat.
- It took Epperson more than 18 years to finally patent his invention. By that time, his own children had taken to calling the treats "popsicles." The new name stuck.
- In 1925, Epperson sold the rights to his popsicle to the John Lowe food company of New York.
- The first commercial popsicles had birch sticks. Today, most sticks are still made of birch.

1 cup frozen blueberries
1 cup baby kale leaves (mature kale is just too "kaley" for this)
2 cups organic purple grape juice

1. In a food processor or high-power blender (such as a VitaMix or BlendTec), blend all ingredients until perfectly liquefied.
2. Pour into ice pop molds or ice cube molds.
3. Freeze until solid.

CHOCOLATE SURPRISE GRANOLA CLUSTERS

MAKES ABOUT 9 CUPS

You guessed it! The "surprise" in this recipe is kale. It's a delicious surprise at that, in an "I can't even taste the kale" kind of way. This is fun to pack in the kids' school lunches to add a touch of sweetness and makes a great "just because" kind of snack. Do not tell anyone

WALNUT LORE

Walnuts are filled with good things—protein, omega-3 fatty acids, vitamin E, and manganese. They benefit the cardiovascular system, the immune system, the skin, and the nervous system. But did you know that only 5.5 percent of American adults eat walnuts at any point in a year? Here are some more fun walnut facts:

- Due to their high polyunsaturated fat content, walnuts are extremely perishable and should be stored in the refrigerator or freezer.
- In the 4th century CE, the Romans introduce walnuts to many European countries, where they have been grown since.
- Walnut oil was once used as lamp oil.
- A 1-ounce serving of walnuts is about 7 shelled walnuts, or 14 walnut halves.
- Walnuts are part of the tree nut family, which includes Brazil nuts, cashews, hazelnuts, macadamia nuts, pecans, pine nuts, and pistachios.
- China is the largest commercial producer of walnuts in the world, with about 360,000 metric tons produced per year.
- The U.S. is the second largest commercial producer of walnuts, with about 294,000 metric tons of production.
- In the U.S., 90 percent of all walnuts are grown in Northern California, most notably, the Sacramento and San Joaquin valleys.
- Turkey, Iran, the Ukraine and Romania are next highest world walnut producers.
- The walnuts grown commercially in the U.S. are known as "English walnuts" because they were first brought to this country on British mercantile ships.
- Black walnuts are native to the U.S.

there is kale in it and they will always ask for seconds (and thirds).

5   dates, pitted and soaked for at least 10 minutes
1   apple or pear, chopped
1   large banana , sliced
2   tablespoons lemon juice
1   tablespoon virgin coconut oil
2   tablespoons cocoa powder
½   teaspoon almond or vanilla extract
4   large leaves of kale, washed, dried, and deribbed
2½ cups old fashioned rolled oats
½   cup unsweetened coconut flakes
½   cup ground oats (you can whir rolled oats in a coffee grinder)
¼   cup milled chia seed (you can whir whole chia seed in a coffee grinder)
½   cup raw sunflower seeds
½   cup walnuts, chopped

1. Preheat the oven to 275°F.
2. In the bowl of a food processor, combine the dates, apple, banana, and lemon juice. Pulse into a smooth puree.
3. Add the coconut oil, cocoa powder, and vanilla. Pulse until incorporated.
4. Add the kale and pulse again until completely incorporated. No kale should be visible.
5. In a large bowl, stir together the rest of the ingredients (oats through walnuts) until well combined. Pour the kale puree over the dry ingredients and stir until evenly coated.
6. Divide the mixture between two or three baking sheets lined with parchment paper and spread evenly over the sheets.
7. Bake for 25 minutes, stir, and bake for another 15 to 20 minutes. Allow to cool completely before transferring to an airtight container and storing in the refrigerator.

COCOA-DUSTED KALE CHIPS
MAKES 2-TO RESERVE SERVINGS

This is another fun, easy and chocolate way to enjoy kale chips. Kids loving helping with this recipe. For a spicy kick, add a sprinkle of chipotle pepper to the cocoa powder.

1   bunch kale, deribbed, washed and perfectly dry
1   teaspoon virgin coconut oil
1   teaspoon agave syrup
2   teaspoons cocoa powder
    Dash salt

1. Preheat an oven to 350°F.
2. Line a non-insulated cookie sheet with parchment paper.
3. In a large bowl, whisk oil and agave until thoroughly combined
4. Add kale to bowl and toss leaves to coat.
5. Sprinkle on cocoa powder and salt, tossing leaves to coat.
6. Arrange kale leaves on one or more baking sheets, so no leaves are touching. Bake for 5 minutes. Turn leaves and continuing baking 10 or more minutes until the edges brown but are not burnt.

DEEP CHOCOLATE-CLOAKED KALE CHIPS

MAKES 2 TO 4 SERVINGS

This unusual recipe is a favorite of true chocoholics. I first tasted it at a party, then again a week later at another party. Knowing a good thing when I taste it, I had to include it here for you to try.

1 *large bunch of kale leaves, deribbed, washed and thoroughly dried*
¼ *cup dark chocolate (preferably 70%), melted*
1 *tsp. virgin coconut oil*
¼ *tsp. sea salt*
Optional: Dash of cinnamon, allspice, or chipotle powder

1. Preheat an oven to 350°F.
2. Line a non-insulated cookie sheet with parchment paper.
3. Place kale leaves in a large bowl and drizzle with oil. Toss leaves to coat.
4. Spread kale evenly onto baking sheet so no leaves are touching
5. Bake for 5 minutes. Turn leaves and continue baking 10 or more minutes until the edges brown but are not burnt
6. Remove from oven. Drizzle with melted dark chocolate. Sprinkle with salt and optional spice.

> **DESSERT CHIPS (KALE-STYLE)**
>
> Dress up your sweet kale chips by dusting them with any of these fun additions:
> - Ground coconut flakes
> - Cinnamon, ginger, allspice, cloves, nutmeg, start anise, cardamom, or a combination of these. A touch of sugar is optional.
> - Finely-milled almond meal or other pulverized nuts
> - Powdered sugar
> - Dried lemon, lime, or orange zest, alone or mixed with powdered sugar

GREEN GODDESS PUDDING

MAKES 2 SERVINGS

This fun recipe is a real kid-pleaser—it's silky, sweet, and chocolate. But a word of very sage advice, from a mom who knows: Do not make this in front of your kids. If they see what's in it, they won't eat it. Which would be unfortunate, as it's packed with omega-3 fatty acids, healthy fats, and all kinds of antioxidants, vitamins, minerals, and fiber.

2 ripe avocados (you want avocados that are
   soft to the touch)
½ cup almond, coconut or rice milk
4 tablespoons cocoa powder (you can use raw
   cacao powder if you have it)
¼ cup agave or mild-tasting honey
¼ cup pureed baby kale (use baby kale for its
   mild flavor)
1 teaspoon vanilla extract
½ teaspoon salt
Optional: chopped nuts and/or saved dark
   chocolate for garnish

1. Add the avocado pulp, milk, cocoa, honey,
kale, vanilla, and salt to the bowl of a food processor. Or use a high-power blender such as
a VitaMix. Process until ingredients are well
blended and the mixture is silky smooth.
2. Ladle into individual pudding cups. If not
eating immediate, cover tightly with food
wrap and keep in the refrigerator.

KALED-UP BOXED MIX BROWNIES

MAKES 4 TO 8 SERVINGS

This is one of those fun "sneaky" recipes
that make the rounds of mommy blogs
and parenting magazines. It's a fun,
delicious way to slide a few tablespoons of
high-impact veggies into resistant kids (and
kid-like adults). Because it uses a boxed
mix, this is fast and easy.

1 box brownie mix (you can use a gluten-free
   mix if you'd like)
¼ cup water
½ cup virgin coconut oil
2 eggs
1 large carrot, steamed until tender (or you can
   use a ¼ cup canned pumpkin puree)
8 kale leaves, deribbed and steamed until tender
Optional: ½ cup chopped nuts, cacao nibs,
   and/or chocolate chips

A NUTTY TOPPER

Sometimes you want to dress up desserts with a cloud of something creamy. A dollop of something rich. Some kind of cream. But for those of us watching our diet, traditional whipped cream
may not be the smartest way to top things off. A great alternative to dairy creams is cashew
cream. To make it, you'll need two cups of raw cashews. Yes, they must be raw. Place them in
the bowl of a high-power blender, such as VitaMix. Or you can use a food processor . Add just
enough water to cover the nuts and process on a high speed for several minutes until the mixture
becomes pale and creamy. Use to top puddings, pies, cake, or sundaes. Store any leftover cream in
a tightly covered container for up to two days in the refrigerator.

WHAT ARE CACAO NIBS?

If you've spent any time in a Whole Foods market, you've probably come across cacao nibs. This little nuggets are partially ground, unprocessed cacao bean. Bitter and intense in taste, nibs are a whole food ingredient with an intense, bitter, chocolate flavor. In other words, nibs don't taste anything like the sugary, milky chocolate of your childhood. Further, small amounts of cacao nibs can be good for you—they're often called a superfood because they are rich in flavonoid antioxidants and the natural vasodilator, theobromine, which helps treat high blood pressure.

1. Pre-heat over to 350°F.

2. Lightly grease an 8- by 8-inch baking pan.

3. Place carrot and kale place the vegetables in a food processor or high-power blender (such as a VitaMix) and puree until perfectly smooth.

4. To the food processor, add water, oil and eggs. Puree until smooth.

5. Add brownie mix to the food processor. Being careful not to overmix, pulse a few times until the batter is blended.

6. If using, add the nuts and/or chocolate chips and pulse twice to blend.

UNDERCOVER KALE COOKIES
MAKES ABOUT 2 DOZEN COOKIES

Sometimes silence really is the best policy. Especially when it comes to giving your kids veggies. If they must have cookies, why not slide in a nourishing range of vitamins, minerals, antioxidants, and omega-3s?

½   cup pureed baby kale

¼   cup unsweetened applesauce

⅓   cup virgin coconut oil

3   eggs

¾   cup sugar

¾   cup packed brown sugar

2   teaspoons vanilla extract

2⅔ cups all-purpose flour or whole wheat
     pastry flour (you can use a mix)

½   cup cocoa

1   teaspoon baking soda

½   teaspoon salt

Optional: Dash cinnamon

Optional: ½ to ¾ cup nuts, chocolate chips,
     or raisins

1. Preheat oven to 350°F.

2. Prepare two baking sheets with parchment or foil.

3. In a large mixing bowl, combine kale puree, applesauce, oil, and eggs. Beat in sugars and vanilla.

4. In a separate mixing bowl, whisk together

flour, cocoa, baking soda, salt, and cinnamon, if using.

5. While mixing, gradually add dry ingredients to kale-applesauce mixture, being careful not to overmix

6. Add in any optional ingredients, stirring just to combine.

7. Cover cookie dough and refrigerate for 2 hours or until slightly firm.

8. Drop dough by rounded teaspoonfuls 2 inches apart onto greased baking sheets. Bake for 8 to 10 minutes, or until edges are browned and cookies are firm.

MAKE YOUR OWN APPLESAUCE

Need applesauce in a pinch? It's quick to make at home. Here's how:

- Take 1 apple. (You can use more if you'd like; you can even use pears. One medium apple will yield about 1 cup of applesauce.)
- Peel apple
- Slice or chop into any size pieces you'd like.
- Place apple into a small saucepan and add 2 or 3 tablespoons of water.
- Cook on medium-low heat until apple breaks down. (Add more water if the pot looks dry; you don't want the apples to scorch.)
- Puree cooked apple and liquid in a food processor or blender until silky smooth.

KALED-UP CHOCOLATE BROWNIES (from scratch)

MAKES 6 TO 10 SERVINGS

Here's another kale-and-carrot brownie recipe, this one from scratch. If someone in your family has trouble with wheat, you can easily use gluten-free oat flour.

3   ounces bittersweet chocolate or chocolate chips
¾   cup carrot or pumpkin puree
¼   cup kale puree
½   cup packed dark brown sugar
¼   cup cocoa powder (unsweetened)
2   tablespoons virgin coconut oil
2   teaspoons vanilla extract
2   large egg whites (or, you can use 1 large whole egg)
¾   cup all-purpose flour (or, you can use the same amount of gluten-free oat flour)
½   teaspoon baking powder
½   teaspoon salt
Optional: ½ cup chopped nuts, cacao nibs and/or chocolate chips

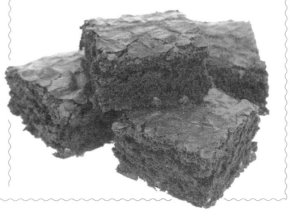

1. Preheat the oven to 350°F.

2. Lightly grease an 8- by 8-inch baking pan.

3. Melt the chocolate over a very low heat or in the microwave 30 seconds at a time.

4. In a large bowl, combine the melted chocolate, carrot puree, kale puree, sugar, cocoa powder, coconut oil, and vanilla in a large bowl. Beat until light and creamy.

5. Whisk in egg whites.

6. In a separate bowl, whisk together flour, baking powder, and salt.

7. Gently fold the dry ingredients into the chocolate mixture, stirring gently just until combined.

8. If using, gently add the nuts and/or chocolate, stirring two or three times only.

9. Pour the batter into prepared pan and bake for 35 to 40 minutes.

10. Cool completely before serving.

COCONUT PRODUCTS DEMYSTIFIED

As people become more and more savvy to coconut's many health benefits, more and more ways to enjoy this superfood appear on health food store shelves. Here is what is currently available:

- Coconut oil is the nutritious oil extracted from fresh coconut meat. Rich in medium-chain fatty acids and phytonutrients, the oil's high smoke point makes it fantastic for cooking. It's also great used as a flavoring and as a hair and skin moisturizer. When buying coconut oil, look for virgin coconut oil, which is obtained through cold-pressing instead of chemical extraction.

- Coconut flour is the finely ground, dried coconut that is left over after extracting coconut oil. Low-carbohydrate, high-fiber, and gluten-free, coconut flour is a darling in the world of wheat-free baking.

- Coconut water is the clear liquid found inside young, green coconuts. Much touted for its amazing ability to replace electrolytes, coconut water is the natural alternative to chemical-laden sports drinks.

- Coconut milk is the meat of the nut blended with water to make a creamy, dairy-like liquid. Once upon a time, all coconut milk came in cans. Now, however, many brands offer cartons of coconut milk in the refrigerated dairy section of your local supermarket or health food store.

- Dried coconut milk is coconut milk that has been dried to a powder, much like dried milk powder. To reconstitute it, simply add milk. It's a handy, shelf-stable ingredient that can be sprinkled directly into soups and curries.

- Coconut cream is what many people call the thickened, creamy looking mixture that sits at the top of a can of coconut milk.

- Cream of coconut goes by many names, including creamed coconut, coconut butter, coconut paste, coconut concentrate and more. This luxurious product is literally a block or jar of thick, shortening-like coconut made from pulverized coconut flesh, oil and all.
- Dried coconut milk is coconut milk that has been dried to a powder, much like dried milk powder. To reconstitute it, simply add milk. It's a handy, shelf-stable ingredient that can be sprinkled directly into soups and curries.
- Desiccated coconut is a baker's favorite! Dried, unsweetened coconut is fine ground for use in cookies, cakes, breads, and other recipes. Don't confuse it with the "sweetened flaked coconut" on store shelves.
- Coconut flakes or chips are related to desiccated coconut, only with bigger flakes.
- Coconut nectar is a low glycemic sweetener made from the sap of coconut trees. Though it does not have a coconuty flavor, it is rich in amino acids, minerals, and vitamins. Use wherever you would use honey or maple syrup.
- Coconut vinegar is similar to apple cider vinegar, except made with coconut water. It is rich in electrolytes and enzymes.
- Coconut aminos are a blend of 17 amino acids, which are harvested from coconut trees and mixed with mineral-rich sea salt. The dark liquid is used as a replacement for soy sauce.
- Coconut yogurt is simply yogurt made with fermented coconut milk instead of fermented cow, sheep, or goat milk. It is a terrific choice for anyone allergic to dairy products.
- Coconut kefir, like its cousin, coconut yogurt, is nothing more than a fermented "yogurt" drink made with coconut milk instead of dairy milk.

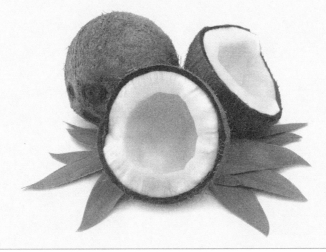

VEGAN COCOA-KALE CUPCAKES

MAKES 12 CUPCAKES

This recipe is based on the famous Wacky Cake recipe that was popular during World War II, a time when eggs and dairy products were scarce. Because it contains no animal ingredients, it is still used heavily in vegan circles. This version goes a step further, adding in a gentle dose of good-for-you kale. If you'd like to use it as a cake, bake it in prepared a 8- by 8-inch or 9- by 9-inch pan.

1½ cups all-purpose flour (you can substitute
     gluten-free all-purpose flour)
¼ cup cocoa
1   cup white sugar
½ teaspoon salt
1   teaspoon baking soda
1   tablespoon white distilled vinegar
⅓ cup virgin coconut oil
1   teaspoon vanilla extract
1   cup cool coffee or water
¼ cup pureed cooked kale

1. Preheat oven to 350°F.
2. Line muffin tin with cupcake liners.
3. In a large bowl, whisk together flour, baking soda, salt, cocoa, and sugar.
4. In a separate bowl, mix together vinegar, oil, vanilla, coffee, and kale.
5. Pour liquid ingredients into dry ingredients and stir just to bend.
6. Fill each muffin tin ¾ full.
7. Bake for 15 minutes or until toothpick inserted comes out clean.
8. Allow to cool in pan for 5 to 10 minutes before removing.

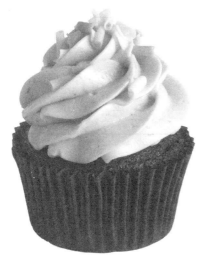
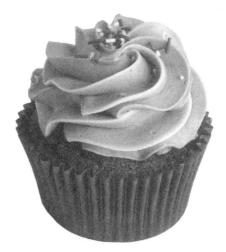

DRESS UP THOSE CUPCAKES

Need to give cupcakes a more formal look or quickly turn muffins into cupcakes? The trick is in the topping. Try one of these ideas:

- Dust with powdered sugar. Go as light or heavy as you'd like.
- Sprinkle vegetable-colored sprinkles (available in specialty stores and health food markets) on to cupcakes when they're partially cooked. Just open up the oven, sprinkle a bit on each cake, close up the oven, and allow the cupcakes to finish baking.
- Frost with whipped cream, drizzle with melted chocolate, or make a simple "mom's" glaze by thinning a cup or two of powdered sugar with coconut milk (or another milk), juice, or water and drizzling on cooled cupcakes.
- Make a powdered sugar buttercream by whipping together one stick of butter, a 1-pound box of powdered sugar, and a splash of vanilla or almond extract. Add 1 or 2 tablespoons of your favorite non-dairy or dairy milk for a smoother consistency.
- Follow the above directions and add 2 tablespoons cocoa powder for chocolate frosting.
- Make a nutbutter frosting with a stick of butter, 1 cup of powdered sugar, 1 teaspoon almond or vanilla extract, ½ cup creamy nutbutter of choice, and a tablespoon or two of your milk of choice. Beat together until smooth.

VEGAN JUICER-PULP MUFFIN

MAKES 12 MINI-MUFFINS

While I don't have conclusive data to back this up, a lot of kale lovers juice regularly. At least I've noticed that my friends who have juicers (and use them regularly—an important distinction), all love kale. So for all of you juicing, kale-loving powerhouses out there, I dedicate this fun cupcake. Dust with powdered sugar or frosting if you'd like.

½ cup juicer pulp (any combination of kale beet/carrot/ginger/pineapple/pear/orange; avoid pulp with any onion-family pulp or anything bitter, such as dandelion)

¼ cup agave syrup

¼ cup virgin coconut oil

¼ cup unsweetened applesauce or pearsauce

1½ cup unbleached flour or gluten-free flour (such as Bob's Red Mill all-purpose gluten-free)

1 teaspoon vanilla extract

1 teaspoon baking soda

½ teaspoon sea salt

½ to 1 teaspoon cinnamon, ginger, allspice, or a mixture of these

Optional: ½ cup chopped dark chocolate or chocolate chips

Optional: ½ cup chopped nuts of choice

1. Pre-heat the oven to 350°F. Lightly grease a mini muffin pan or line with paper muffin cups.

2. In a large bowl, add the juicer pulp, making sure to remove any large pieces.

3. To the juicer pulp, add the agave, coconut oil, applesauce, and vanilla. Stir to combine.

4. In a separate bowl, whisk together flour, baking soda, salt, and chosen spice. Add the optional chocolate and/or nuts and whisk again.

5. Add dry ingredients to pulp mixture. Mix gently with a silicone spatula or wooden spoon until just combined. (The batter will be thick.)

6. Transfer the batter to the mini muffin pan and bake for 10 to 12 minutes. A knife inserted in the center should come out clean when they're done.

7. Allow to cool for 10 minutes before removing from the pan. When cool, dust with powdered sugar or decorate with your favorite frosting.

WHAT TO DO WITH THE PULP?

More and more people than ever are discovering the joys of juicing. Creating and drinking home-pressed juice is not only fun, it is one of the healthiest things you can do for your body. But what to do with all that pulp? Most of us toss it into the compost heap, but you'll be glad to know that it's perfectly usable. Here are some ideas that'll use up between ¼ and ½ cup of fruit or veggie pulp:

- Puree it into creamy soups.
- Add it to marinara and other pasta sauces. To ensure a smooth, kid-friendly finish, give the sauce whir in a blender before serving.
- Add to a blender-made smoothie.
- Use as a filler for meatloaf, meatballs, shepherd's and cottage pie, and other ground meat recipes.
- Add to crab cakes, veggie burgers, potato pancakes, and similar foods.
- Tuck into baked goods, including muffins, tea breads, and cakes.

WICKED KALE CUPCAKES

MAKES 24 CUPCAKES

This is a traditional, Devils Food-style cupcake, which can also be baked in two 8-inch or 9-inch pans … should you have a hankering for a luscious layer cake. If you're out of kale, you can use spinach puree or even beet puree.

2   *cups sugar*
1¾   *cups flour*
¾   *cup cocoa*
1½   *teaspoons baking powder*
1½   *teaspoons baking soda*
2   *eggs*
1   *cup dairy or non-dairy milk of choice*
¼   *cup virgin coconut oil*
¼   *cup pureed kale*
1   *cup boiling coffee or water*

1. Heat oven to 350°F.
2. Line cupcake pans with paper liners (or grease and flour 2 cake pans).
3. In a large bowl, whisk together sugar, flour, cocoa, baking powder, and baking soda.
4. In the bowl of an electric mixer on medium speed, beat together eggs, milk, oil, and kale for 2 minutes. Stir in boiling coffee or water.
5. Add dry ingredients to the liquid ingredients and beat for a minute, until combined. The batter will be very thin; don't worry, all is well!
6. Pour batter into muffin cups, filling each ¾ full.
7. Bake 20 to 25 minutes or until a wooden toothpick inserted in the center comes out clean.

WHAT THE DEVIL?

Devil's Food cakes begin appearing in the United States in the early 1900s. These were chocolate cakes that featured a thin, coffee-infused batter with a measure of shredded beets (think of a carrot cake, only made with beets and chocolate). The beets not only added body and moisture to the cake, they infused it with its devilish crimson hue. The name Devil's Food was originally a play on the white Angel's Food cakes that appeared a few years earlier.

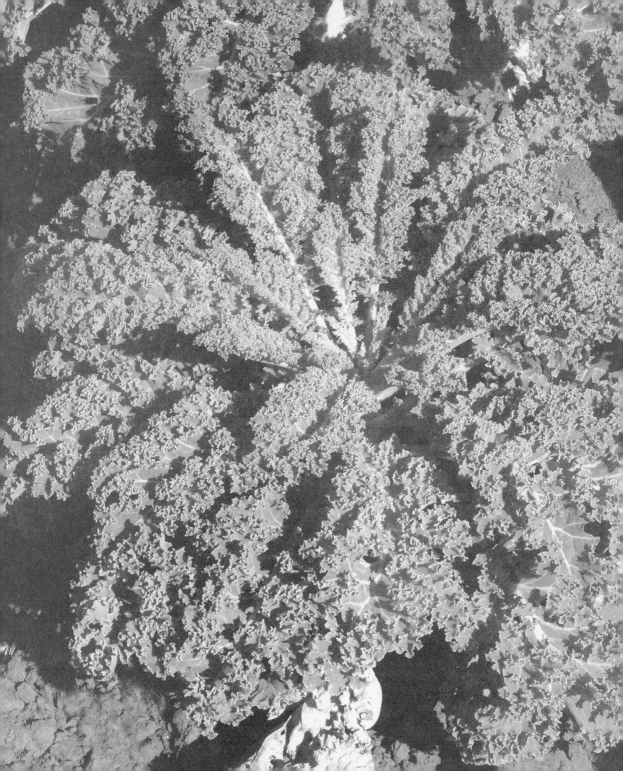

CHAPTER 9

FREQUENTLY ASKED QUESTIONS

When you have an ingredient as powerful—with as many wide-ranging benefits—as kale, there are bound to be questions. Here are some of the kale questions I am asked over and over again.

NUTRIENTS AND BENFITS

What minerals does kale have?

Manganese, copper, tryptophan, calcium potassium, iron, magnesium, and phosphorous.

What vitamins does kale have?

Vitamins A, B1, B2, B3, B6, C, E, K, and folate.

What else does kale contain?

Insoluble fiber, protein, glucosinolates, flavonoids, carotenoids, omega-3 fatty acids, and chlorophyll.

I've heard kale has an incredible amount of vitamin K. What, exactly, does vitamin K do in the body?

One cup of cooked kale contains 1062.10 micrograms of vitamin K—or 1327.6 percent of your daily requirement for the nutrient. This under-celebrated vitamin helps the body's fight inflammation. Vitamin K is also needed for proper bone formation and blood clotting and is used by the body to help transport calcium.

What are glucosinolates?

The scientific definition of a glucosinolate is a class of organic compounds that contain sulfur and nitrogen and are derived from glucose and an amino acid. Known for their anticancer properties, the glucosinolates found in kale are glucobrassicin, glucoraphanin, gluconasturtiian, glucopaeolin, and sinigrin.

When you chew kale, you release these glucosinolates into your body, where they activate the body's own detoxification systems, slowing cancer cell growth and assisting in DNA repair.

What are flavonoids?

Once known collectively as Vitamin P, flavonoids are antioxidants that are responsible for giving blue, green, and green-yellow plants their coloration. As of this writing, researchers have identified 45 different flavonoids in kale.

They are also known for combating allergens, viruses, and carcinogens, as well as having anti-inflammatory, anti-microbial, anti-cancer, and anti-diarrheal properties.

What are carotenoids?

Like flavonoids, carotenoids are antioxidants that are responsible for giving plants (golden yellow, orange, and red plants) their coloration. Carotenoids are widely celebrated for immune-protecting and immune-system-strengthening-abilities. Scientists haven't yet identified the exact number of individual carotenoids in kale.

How much omega-3 fatty acid does kale have?

A one-cup serving of kale contains 0.13 grams of omega-3 fatty acids. While there are foods, such as chia, salmon, and walnuts, which contain higher levels of omega-3 fatty acids, kale does contain a respectable amount.

What is an essential fatty acid?

Essential fatty acids are so called because they cannot be synthesized in the body; it is therefore essential they be obtained from foods. Omega-6 and omega-3 are the essential fatty acids for humans and other animals. They are precursors of powerful hormones that affect many biological processes; they help maintain healthy skin, and are involved in cholesterol metabolism.

Is one fatty acid better than another?

The only one that is essential is ALA (alpha linolenic acid), the type of omega-3 found in kale. DHA and EPA, which come from marine sources, are not essential omega-3 fatty acids since they can be synthesized by the body (converted from ALA).

What is the appropriate omega-6 to omega-3 ratio?

The ideal ratio is from 1:1 to 3:1. During our evolutionary period, humans ate an omega-6/omega-3 ratio of 1:1. Modern diets are very rich in omega-6, derived primarily from vegetable and animal fats. Typically, today's diets provide ratios that are greater than 15:1 omega-6 to omega-3. This imbalance increases the risk of coronary heart disease and also heightens the body's natural inflammatory processes.

How to omega-6 and omega-3 fatty acids compare?

In general omega-3's are anti-inflammatory, whereas omega-6's are just the opposite, the promote inflammation.

Can kale help me lose weight?

Yes! Kale is high in insoluble fiber and low in calories. A one-cup serving of steamed kale contains about 36 calories and boasts 10.4 percent of your daily's need for fiber. Eating fiber-rich foods gives you a pleasant feeling of satiety or fullness—if you feel full, you'll be less likely to overeat.

What is the difference between soluble and insoluble fiber?

Insoluble fiber does not swell or dissolve in

water and passes through the digestive system in much the same way it entered the system. Insoluble fiber is great for intestinal health, and helps with constipation, hemorrhoids, and colorectal cancer. Soluble fiber is found in kale, peas, beans, lentils, oatmeal, and the pectin of fruit.

Soluble fiber is "swellable" in water. When mixed with liquid, it forms a gel-like substance and swells. It is great for moderating blood glucose levels and lowering cholesterol. Most of the soluble fiber humans currently eat comes from the outer layer of cereal grains.

Is kale good for persons with arthritis?

Kale is very good for people with arthritis or any type of joint pain, because it is high in omega-3 fatty acid and antioxidants, all of which are powerful anti-inflammatory agents. Research has also indicated that intake of vitamin C-rich foods (such as kale) protects against inflammatory arthritis.

I've heard kale is great for diabetics. Why?

The fiber in kale helps slow the rate of carbohydrates, conversion into sugar, thus helping to maintain healthy blood sugar levels.

I'm looking for a way to get more easily assimilated minerals into my diet. Can kale help?

Yes! Kale contains an impressive dose of several minerals, including 27 percent of your recommended daily allowance of manganese, 10 percent of copper, and 9.4 percent of calcium, plus potassium, iron, magnesium, and phosphorous.

I heard Dr. Oz say that kale may decrease the risk of Alzheimer's disease. How?

One of contributing factor in Alzheimer's disease is inflammation, specifically, inflammation in the brain and nervous system. Kale is rich in folate, vitamin E, and omega-3 fatty acids, three anti-inflammatory ingredients which Dr. Oz says can reduce Alzheimer's risk by up to one-third.

GROWING KALE

I would love to try growing kale in my backyard, but I live in a cooler climate. Is that a problem?

Actually, it's a benefit. At least where kale is concerned. (Hot weather turns kale bitter.) It prefers cool temperatures and will be sweetened by a touch of frost. It will start to turn bitter and become tough in temperatures over 80°F. (This is why my kids won't eat kale from California—they can taste the difference between cool-weather and warm-climate kale.)

Kale's favorite soil temperature is 55 to 65°F. If planting in colder climates, wait until spring and directly seed as soon as the soil can be worked and the soil temperature is at least 45°F.

What kind of soil does kale prefer?

Kale isn't a fussy plant—it gives so much and asks so little in return! It will grow in most soil, but like most veggies, it loves loamy, well-drained soil with a pH between 5.5 and 6.8. If yours isn't that, start about two weeks before planting and work in a few shovelfuls of manure into the soil. Break up any large, hard clumps to improve drainage.

How long does it take kale to grow from seed to a fully mature plant?

Anywhere from 55 to 65 days, depending upon the variety of seed, where you live, and the temperatures there.

Does kale like sun or shade?

In more Northern climates, kale prefers full or near-full sun. In warmer climates it can tolerate filtered or partial sun.

How much room does kale need in the garden?

Space each plant about 12 inches apart, in rows that are 2 feet distant from each other.

Does kale need to be covered in the winter?

Not if you live where winters are mild. If your average winter temperatures are in the low 30s°F or lower, cover the plants with a layer of mulch. You should be able to harvest into the cold weather months by simply removing any outer leaves you'd like to use.

How do I harvest kale?

Cut away from the outer leaves. The plant will continue to grow as long as the center leaves are intact.

The easiest way to remove the leaves is with garden shears, though many gardeners use the "grab, twist, and break-off" method of leaf harvesting.

Can I grow kale in pots?

Yes. In fact it grows really well in pots, window boxes, and other containers. Plus, kale's gorgeous foliage make it the perfect "functional ornamental" (in other words, something that looks AND tastes fabulous!). For best results, choose a 6-inch container or larger.

To grow, choose regular kale (not "ornamental kale") seeds and sow ½ inch deep, spaced 3 inches apart. The best time to plant is spring. To extend your growing and harvesting seasons, you can move pots of kale into shade when the weather begins to get warm.

Will kale grow indoors?

It will, but you probably won't get the lush, fat leaves of garden-grown kale; without natural sunlight, kale grows exceedingly slowly and spindly indoors. A pot outside a windowsill may be a better choice.

I'm thinking of growing several varieties of kale and am looking for ideas. Which ones do you like?

I love Lacinto kale (also known as Nero, dinosaur, or Tuscan kale). I find it the most flavorful variety. Being my favorite, I would definitely include it. That said, it is the slowest grower of the varieties and it doesn't over-winter as well as the others. So you'll want to mix things up and choose at least one other variety.

Red Russian and White Russian varieties love the cold and are super vigorous. They also have a sweeter taste that a lot of people prefer.

Lastly, if you're looking for something pretty to dress things up a bit, there are several varieties of curly leaf kale with bright purple or red-tinted leaves. I like the Scarlet curly leaf kale. It's gorgeous!

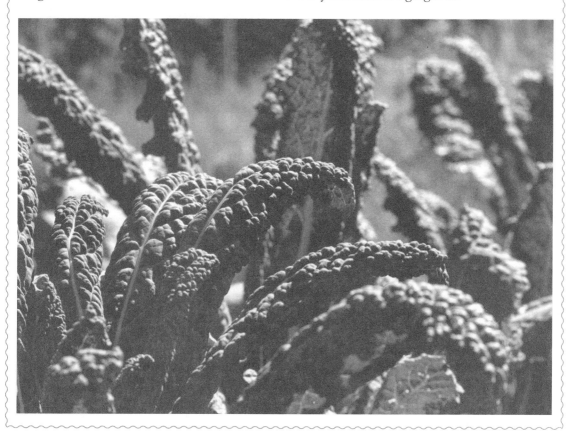

How much kale should I plant for a family of three?

It really depends on how much kale you use. If you juice it, make smoothies with it, snack on homemade kale chips, and use it in several dishes a week, you'll want more than someone who only eats it every once-in-awhile. A good rule of thumb: Those who eat kale three or four times a week should plant five plants per person. Unless you like to freeze veggies, in which case you should double that amount.

Do deer and rabbits like kale?

Yes, they do. And so do chipmunks, gophers, mice, moles, opossums, raccoons rats, skunks, turtles, voles, and woodchucks. You may want to build a fence around your garden, then plant a few stray kale plants as far away from your plot as possible, to lure animal visitors away from your veggies!

Are there any helpful plants that should be planted near kale to help protect it from pests?

Known as companion planting, the practice of planting certain plants near each other is a fascinating and surprisingly ancient gardening trick. Many plants will dwarf other plants, casting them in unwanted shadow. Others attract certain pests, which could kill a neighbor. On the other hand, one plant may lure ladybugs, which will them go to work devouring the aphids on a next-door plant. Some might give off nitrogen or other helpful substances into the soil, which can enhance everyone's growth.

Kale (and its cruciferous cousins) does well with beets, celery, dill, Swiss chard, lettuce, spinach, onions, and potatoes planted nearby. Thyme, is a particularly well-suited companion which helps repel the cabbage worm.

Are there any plants that kale should *not* be planted near?

While kale gets along with most veggies, it doesn't do so well with pole beans, which overwhelm shorter kale plants and block necessary sunlight.

COOKING WITH KALE

I love cooking with kale, but I feel guilty throwing away the rib and stem. Is there anything I can do with them?

You could mince them and throw them into long-simmering soups and stews. If you have a powerful blender, such as VitaMix or BlendTec, you can whir them with broth, garlic, a handful of green peas, and half an avocado for quick nourishing soup. Or—and this is my favorite way—you can run them through the juicer. They are filled with liquid and add powerful nutrients to your morning glass of green juice.

Every time I make kale chips they come out soggy. What am I doing wrong?

You're probably oversaturating the leaves with oil. You need very little oil to make fantastic kale chills. In fact, the less the better. Try using less than a tablespoon on a full bunch of kale. You want to barely coat the leaves.

Every time I make kale chips they come out too soft. What am I doing wrong?
The kale leaves must be perfectly dry before you toss them with oil and salt. If you notice any moisture on your kale leaves, toss them in a salad spinner and wick off all remaining liquid. Once they are bone-dry, you can proceed with the recipe.

Every time I make kale chips they come out tough and chewy. What am I doing wrong?
You may be undercooking them. The darker varieties of kale, such as Lacinto kale (also known as dinosaur or Nero kale) can be quite dark in color. Because it is difficult to tell whether the edges of such deeply-colored leaves are browned, it's easy to remove them from the oven too early (or too late!).

You want the edges of the leaves to be lightly brown. If it's easier for you, try a batch using the lighter-colored curly leaf kale.

My kale chips take forever to cook. Or they cook unevenly. Why?
Be sure to give your leaves plenty of space on the baking sheet! When leaves are bunched on top of each other, they don't cook evenly, nor do they have a chance to get thoroughly cooked, with the crisp finish we expect from out kale chips!

My sautéed kale always tastes so bitter. Is there something I can do to soften the bitterness?
Yes, you can blanch the kale before sautéing. You'll find instructions on page 12, but in a nutshell, blanching involves plunging kale (or other vegetables) into vigorously boiling water, then immediately removing it. This "pre-cooking" often removes bitterness from kale and other brassica-family veggies. When you're ready to sauté it, chop, add to the pan, and season as per your recipe.

Sometimes my kale takes so long to cook. Why?
The older the kale leaves, the longer they'll take to cook. Kale that is harvested young has less fiber and becomes tender much more quickly when cooked, than leaves that are more mature and larger.

When it comes to kale, I like to say "you cook it until it's done." This could mean 10 minutes, 15 minutes, or even 20 minutes.

What to do with an abundance of kale?
I have a few bunches of kale and don't want to eat all of it at once. What should I do with them?

Blanch them (see page 12). You can sauté whatever portion you'd like to use within five days. Try olive oil and garlic and dress with any sauce (salsa, curry, pesto, salsa, marinara, etc.). Freeze anything you can't eat within five days.

What's the best kale to use in my morning smoothies? I find the curly kale I'm using now doesn't break down well.

We drink a lot of green smoothies in my household and here's what I do: I save the mature kale leaves (regardless of the variety) for the juicer and use baby kale leaves for the blender-made smoothies. The baby kale leaves break down quicker and much more thoroughly. Try it!

Do you have a favorite kale variety?

I'll preface this with: I adore kale. All varieties! Put a bunch in front of me and I instantly want to make something with it. I love the way it looks, the way it feels, and the way it tastes. I love how strong and energized I feel when I eat it regularly, and how great my skin looks. But I do have a favorite. It's Lacinto kale. I adore the deep green color and the nubbly texture. And I find it easier to cut than the curly varieties. But like I said, I certainly wouldn't turn away any curly kale leaf that crossed my path.

HISTORY AND BACKGROUND
Where does kale come from?

There are conflicting opinions about this. Some researchers feel kale was first eaten in the Mediterranean, where it was a favorite of the Romans, who carried it north. Others are just as sure that it originated in Asia Minor and was brought to Europe by Celtic nomads. Wherever it began, we do know is that it quickly spread to Europe and then the British Isles, where it became an important part of those populations' diets.

How old is kale?

It is believed that early kale—which grew wild and had smaller, slimmer leaves than to-day's kale—was being eaten before 600 BCE, when it first appeared in Europe.

Is it true that cabbage is a new form of kale?

In a way, yes. Brussels' sprouts, broccoli, cabbage, cauliflower, collard, and kohlrabi are all descendents of wild kale.

Is kale native to North America?

No. It was first brought across the Atlantic in the late 1600s by settlers from the British Isles.

Why is kale associated with Northern Europe?

Kale was one of the most important foodstuffs in Europe until the arrival of the potato. It was consumed at every meal, and most homes kept an enclosed kale garden (known in the British Isles as a kale yard).

What is a Kale Queen?

Kale Queens are a uniquely German phenomenon. In the northwestern cities of Germany, it is popular to partake in "kale tours."

These involve kale festivals where people sample various kale dishes, judge kale plants, drink beer, talk kale, and crown some lucky young woman "Kale Queen."

I've heard there was a literature movement in Scotland that had to do with kale. What does kale have to do with literature?

In Scotland, most homes had what was known as a "kailyard," an enclosed garden used for growing kale and other vegetables. Kale was so important to the Scotts, that the name for dinner was the same as the name for the vegetable.

The Kailyard School of literature showed Scottish life in a sentimental, romantic light. Popular in the 1890s, one of the most loved books of this movement was *Beside the Bonnie Brier Bush* by Ian MacLaren.

CHOOSING AND STORING KALE

How do I choose the freshest kale?

If you want the absolute freshest kale available, you'll want to grow it and pick it yourself. If that's not an option for you, head to the nearest farmer's market and pick up some locally grown kale. Chances are, locally grown kale was picked only a day or two earlier.

What you don't want to do is buy kale that has been shipped across country (or flown in from another country). If you live in Maryland, you don't want to buy kale that has been picked in California, packed onto a truck, driven five days across country to a grocery store in your town, unpacked, stacked in the grocery store produce department and allowed to sit for several days before you go shopping, see it and purchase it. Not very fresh, is it?

An easy way to tell if kale is old is color. The curly leaf kale varieties in particular tend to yellow as they age. In past-prime kale, leaves and stalks get dried out and wilted, or wet and slimy. These are all signs that you should not buy it.

Kale seems so hardy. Does it lose nutrients after it's been picked?

It does. Leafy greens (such as kale) are particularly susceptible to nutrient loss. One recent study showed that kale lost 89 percent of its vitamin C when left at 70°F for two days after picking. Freezing helps retain nutrients. That same study found that when kale that was stored just above freezing, only lost 5 percent of its vitamin C.

To help slow nutrient loss, start with the freshest kale available and use or refrigerate as soon as possible.

Lastly, vitamins, antioxidants, and enzymes are most likely to die in storage; minerals, fiber and protein are not greatly affected.

My kale looks wilted. How can I revive it?

You can. But before I tell you how, I must say this: If your kale has gone limp, a portion of its nutrients has probably significantly diminished.

To revive wilted kale, soak the leaves in ice water. The cold water hydrates and plumps up tired vegetable fibers.

How long can I keep kale in my fridge?

This will depend a bit upon how fresh your kale is—was it grown nearby and was it picked in the last couple of days? If you're unsure of where your kale comes from, or how old it was when you bought it, try to use it within three days or purchase. You can go up to five days if your kale was fresh-picked. For longer storage, blanch kale leaves (see page 12) and freeze.

Does kale freeze well?

Yes! It freezes beautifully. Blanch leaves first (see page 12), then store in an airtight container in the freezer.

KALE AND SAFETY

Could kale cause problems in people with diverticulitis? I have heard conflicting advice from various doctors.

Diverticulosis is a condition characterized by the formation of small pouches, or diverticulae, in your large intestine. At one time, it was widely believed that high-fiber foods, such as kale, would get trapped in these small pouches, aggravating the condition. Newer research has found that kale can actually be especially beneficial to those with diverticulitis and other related conditions, such as Irritable Bowel Syndrome. Talk to your health provider before adding kale to your diet, but it has been suggested that the fiber in kale can help heal diverticulitis by creating regularity. Further, kale is extremely high in vitamin K, which has been shown to heal intestinal tissue.

I've heard that people who have had kidney stones should avoid kale. Why?

Oxalates. These naturally-occurring substances are produced by the body. Oxalates are also found in some animal and plant food, including leafy green veggies like spinach, chard, and kale. Individuals with larger amounts of oxalates in their bodies may be at risk for kidney stones when they eat foods containing oxalates. That's because these molecules bind together to create kidney stones.

One of my mother's friends said she couldn't eat kale because of her goiter. What is a goiter and why would kale affect it?

A goiter is simply a visibly enlarged thyroid gland, which can occur when the thyroid gland isn't functioning properly. They can be caused by an autoimmune disorder, such as Hashimoto's Disease or Graves Disease, which affect the thyroid gland. Another cause is an iodine deficiency. The primary activity of the thyroid gland is to concentrate iodine from the blood to make thyroid hormone. The gland cannot make enough thyroid hormone if it does not have enough iodine. Therefore, individuals with iodine deficiency will become hypothyroid.

At one time, goiters were quite commonplace. While they remain common in many parts of the world, today, however, they are very rare in First World countries, most of which use iodized salt. In fact, the first time I ever heard the word goiter was on a *Seinfeld* episode.

So what does this have to do with kale?

Cruciferous vegetables such as kale, cabbage, Brussels sprouts, broccoli, and cauliflower contain natural chemicals called goitrogens (goiter producers) that can interfere with thyroid hormone synthesis. While the goitrogens in these foods are inactivated by cooking, there are physicians who suggest that people with goiters avoid these veggies. It sounds as if your mother's friend may have one of these doctors. As always, you want to consider your health-care practitioner's advice when choosing food to keep you healthy.

Is it safe to eat conventionally grown kale? I've heard it is grown with a lot of pesticides.

Several different types of bugs—including aphids, grasshoppers, cabbage loopers, cabbageworm, cutworms, and flea beetles—love kale. This means large swaths of kale can be a Mecca for these bugs. To keep their crops from being decimated by these hungry pests, many farmers rely on conventionally-grown kale, which is typically sprayed with pesticides such as Metam potassium, 1,3-Dichloropropene, Malathion, DCPA, and several others.

Because many of these pesticides cannot be fully removed by cleaning, and because kale cannot be peeled, there are traces of these chemicals on conventionally-grown kale.

Organic farmers have a few tricks up their sleeves to help keep pests at bay. This includes spreading out kale, so insects don't settle into a field of kale, moving easily from plant to plant to plant. They also have natural pest management methods, such as soapy water and neem oil (yes, even on an agricultural scale!).

So my answer is this: If you can easily buy, organic, do. Yet do not forgo kale if you can't buy organic: It is just too healthy to pass up, even when grown conventionally. Simply wash it in soapy water or in water with a teaspoon of baking soda to remove as much of the pesticides as possible.

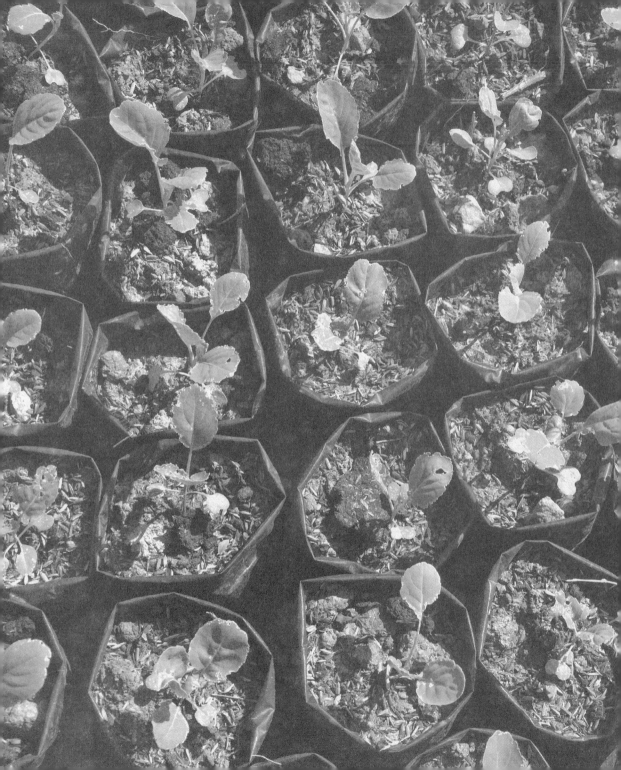

CHAPTER 10

KALE-GROWING GUIDE

Kale is easy to grow and fun to harvest. Plus, nothing tastes like salad that's been made with greens harvested just minutes before. There are all kinds of fun varieties to try, and growing your own food is one of the most environmentally friendly things you can do for the planet. And it's an easy challenge for all you do-it-yourself types.

Ready to give it a go? Good! Let's head out to the garden!

WHAT KALE LIKES

Not too rich, not too sandy. Not too wet, not too dry. Not too fine, not too rocky. Not to hot, not too shady. Kale likes things just so!

Choose a spot that gets between two and six hours of direct sun a day. Kale may not like heat, but it does like light. Kale also prefers loamy, well-drained, and moist (not too soggy, not too dry) soil. If this is your first time planting kale, deeply prepare the soil, mixing in compost or manure. Some people add some limestone to the soil, saying it encourages lusher growth.

Lightweight, sandy soils and heavy clay soils will impact the health and the flavor of kale, though kale may still grow in these soils. (For you gardeners out there who like to use gardening terms, go for a soil pH of 5.5 to 6.8.)

KALE LIKES THINGS COOL

There are some veggies out there, such as tomatoes and peppers, who just adore the heat of summer. Kale is not one of these! It appreciates cool temperatures, moderate sun, a frost or two to make the leaves taste sweeter. Temperatures from 20 to 65°F are best, and a few freezing or below-zero temperature days are just fine.

When growing kale, think cool and bright. If you've got mild summers that won't scorch heat-sensitive kale, go ahead and plant your seeds in the spring; they'll grow over the summer for a fall harvest. You'll have kale just in time for Halloween and Thanksgiving! If your area has intense summers and gentle winters, aim for an autumn planting. The kale can grow through the winter for a spring harvest.

> ### HOW MUCH TO GROW
>
> One seed packet will give you enough kale to feed a family of four to six people.

PURCHASE THE SEEDS

Check out any reputable garden center, plant seller, seed catalog or online seed store and you'll find dozens of different varieties of kale, each more gorgeous and intriguing than the next.

ARE YOU IN THE ZONE?

For help on choosing planting times, it helps to know what agricultural zone you're in. In the United States—and in most other countries—the government's agricultural department separates the country into planting zones. Each zone represents a micro-climate which works best for a number of specific plants. In the United States, zones 5 through 9 are particularly kale-friendly. For more information on USDA plant hardiness zones, visit: **www.planthardiness.ars.usda.gov/**.

Most of us have favorite types. Some of us love the curly "Scotch-style" kales, others enjoy the red "Russian-style" leaves. While others still like the unfrilled, narrow, "Tuscan" varieties. My advice: Head to a store or a site, check out what's available, matching interesting-looking varieties with your needs and climate. Choose one or more suitable varieties and experiment. Playing with different varieties of a plant is what makes gardening so creative and fun. Much more fun than heading to the supermarket and buying the lone kale variety sitting in the produce department.

PREPARE THE SITE

One of the most important things you can do when planting anything, kale included, is prepare the soil. Start by removing weeds, which can later choke and kill your young

KALE COMPANIONS

Companion planting is the practice of using plants' natural preferences to create a healthier garden that needs less human and chemical intervention. It works by planting situating certain plants near other plants which can help each other. Many companion vegetables, herbs, and fruits help to deter pests, which helps to decrease the amount of pesticides and effort it takes to keep your garden pest-free. Companion planting frequently also increases the yields of the plants so you get more food from the same space.

Kale's best garden buddies are beets, celery, cucumbers, dill, garlic, hyssop, lettuce, mint, nasturtium, onions, potatoes, rosemary, sage, spinach, and Swiss chard. Plan on planting these in rows next to each other or even alternating plants within a row. If you can, keep kale away from its least favorite companions, which are beans, strawberries, and tomatoes.

KALE IN A CONTAINER

Maybe you don't have access to a single patch of dirt. Or maybe you just don't want to fuss with tilling, sowing, and thinning. Fortunately for you, kale grows beautifully outdoors in pots. (It doesn't do so well indoors in pots—it grows spindly and pale.) Follow the same directions as you would for growing kale in the garden, with these adjustments:

- Choose a pot that's at least 8-inches deep and 8-inches wide. Go larger if you want larger plants.
- Because kale likes cooler temperatures, opt for early spring or autumn planting.
- Fill the pot ⅔ of the way up with soil, then top it off with rich compost mixed with a small amount of organic fertilizer. Check your fertilizer for mixing instructions.
- Plant one or two kale seeds in the center of the pot, about a ½-inch deep.
- Place the pot somewhere where the soil temperature is at least 45°F and no more than 65°F—75°F is ideal. This is called the germination period and if you'd like, you can move the pot or pots into a greenhouse or even indoors next to a window.
- In five to eight days, you'll see the plants break through the soil. Move the pots, weather permitting, outdoors to a spot that gets no warmer than 75°F. Kale doesn't like hot temperatures.
- Water a few times a week. You want soil to be slightly moist. Not parched and not wet.

CAN I EAT IT?

A popular winter flour in the East—New Yorkers will recognize it from outdoor flower beds—ornamental kale is, indeed, edible. It has a mellower flavor and tender texture than garden kale. Ornamental kale was first cultivated commercially during the 1980s in California. Oftentimes referred to as salad savoy, its leaves may either be pale or deep green, white, or purple, and its stalks coalesce to form a loosely knit head.

kale plants. Remember to remove weeds from the roots so they won't regrow.

Next, break up the soil with a rake or hoe, diminishing large clods of earth. Work in a manure-enriched compost, leaf mold, peat moss or a mixture of these. For you soil testers out there, kale's favorite pH is about 6.5, so if your soil is acidic you can add crushed calcium limestone or shell limestone to sweeten it.

KALE: PREVENTING DISEASE

Kale is a hardy plant, one that doesn't need a lot of special attention. That said, kale can succumb to one of several diseases or pests. To ensure that doesn't happen, follow these preventative measures:

- Inspect plants a few times a week. If you notice a problem, you can address it immediately.
- Water the soil rather than the plant. Wet plants are more susceptible to diseases than dry ones.
- Also, avoid splashing soil onto the plants when you water.
- Clean your tools thoroughly before moving from one part of the garden to another or keep separate sets of tools in different parts of the garden.
- If you're walking or working in an infested or sick part of the garden, do not visit your kale plants until you've washed your hands, changed your clothes, and cleaned the dirt off your shoes. Bits of soil or pests can travel from one part of the garden to another on your hands, clothing, or your shoes.
- Introduce ladybugs and other beneficial insects that are adept at wiping out aphid infestations.

USING SEEDLINGS

As you immerse yourself in the world of gardening, you'll hear the words "seedlings" and "transplants" bandied about. Here's what these terms refer to: Instead of planting seeds directly into the ground, you first plant them in small pots, allow them to germinate and begin growing in a warm, safe place. You then transplant the young plant directly into the ground.

It sounds like a lot of extra work, doesn't it? But there's a reason you may want to use seedlings: It allows you to get a jump on the growing season. By starting plants indoors, you can get right to the business of growing. Once the weather has warmed up a bit and soil temperatures become toasty enough for plants to thrive, you can plug your seedlings directly into the ground. (Try not to look smugly at those gardeners who will be just starting to directly sow their seeds in the ground.)

PLANT THE SEEDS

You've got your seeds, the soil is prepared, the ground is warming—it's time to get planting! Sow kale seeds in rows for easy harvest. Bury seeds ¼- to ½-inch deep, 1 inch apart, and make sure rows are spaced at least 18 inches apart from each other. Kale germinates easily in coolish or barely warm soil temperatures with even moisture.

THIN THE SEEDLINGS

Thinning is the act of removing plants. I know, it sounds counterintuitive, doesn't it? But it's an important way to ensure each kale plant has the space it needs, and the access to water and sun it needs, to grow to its full potential. To thin kale seedlings, wait until the young plants have three true leaves. This may be between two-and-a-half to four weeks. Remove the weakest-looking of the plants, leaving the strongest seedlings about 8 inches to a full foot apart. Don't toss the removed seedlings! You can add them to salads or stir-fries, replant them in a pot or a different part of the garden, or give them to a friend or family member to plant in their garden.

CULTIVATE THE KALE

Kale isn't fussy, but it does like to stay moist. So the nicest thing you can do is to keep your kale watered. Not overwatered, not soggy, not soaked. Just lightly moist. Moisture, along with cooler temperatures, is the secret to sweet, crisp kale leaves—they get bitter when exposed to above 85°F temperatures or allowed to dry out.

To further support your kale, remove yellowing leaves whenever you see them, make sure there is earth packed around the lower stems, and think about feeding kale with a scattering of compost or manure or fish emulsion at least once during the growing period. While kale plants do love nippy temperatures, if it's winter, consider covering your plants with mulch or hay to keep them productive.

HARVEST THE KALE

For most regular, non-dwarf kale varieties, harvest happens about two months after planting. Or when they reach 15 to 20 cm in length. Once the plant reaches maturity, you can simply chop the plant off at the base of the stalk. I like to wait after the first frost before harvesting—the leaves are so much more sweet and tasty.

But you have another fun option—a bit of a kale-growing secret: Kale can be treated as a cut-and-come-again plant, meaning you can continually cut small leaves for salad or other dishes as needed these leaves will replace themselves. Use a sharp knife or shears and clip leaves at the stalk. You can continue to clip and come back, clip and come back until the plant puts out flowers, usually in the warmer months.

RESOURCES

HISTORY BOOKS

100 Vegetables and Where They Came From
By William Woys Weaver
(Algonquin Books, 2000)
A cornucopia of vegetables and stories from around the world—from Argentina to Zimbabwe, from Australia to the United States.

How Carrots Won the Trojan War: Curious (but True) Stories of Common Vegetables
By Rebecca Rupp (Storey Publishing, 2011)
A collection of little-known stories about the origins, legends, and historical significance of 23 of the world's most popular vegetables.

Vegetable Gardening the Colonial Williamsburg Way: 18th-Century Methods for Today's Organic Gardeners
By Wesley Greene (Rodale, 2012)
A guide to traditional—and still relevant—methods and advice for planting and tending kale and other traditional vegetable favorites.

Vegetables: A Biography
By Evelyne Bloch-Dano
(University of Chicago Press, 2012)
Through detailed biographies of eleven different vegetables, Evelyne Bloch-Dano explores the world of vegetables in all its facets, from science and agriculture to history, culture, and, of course, cooking.

GARDENING BOOKS

Brooklyn Botanical Guide for a Greener Planet, Edible Gardens
By Elizabeth Peters
(Brooklyn Botanic Garden, 2011)
Learn about everything from easy-to-grow annuals to long-fruiting perennials, this encyclopedia of edible plants offers colorful profiles highlighting each plant's ornamental attributes, origins, use as food, and cultivation requirements.

Gardening by Cuisine
By Patti Moreno (Sterling, 2013)
Even urban dwellers, with little more than a balcony or tiny backyard or windowsill, can grow their own food, thanks to Patti Moreno's groundbreaking gardening guide! Moreno, host of the most popular garden videos on the Web, has devised a unique plan for creating low-maintenance organic "cuisine gardens."

The Girl's Guide to Growing Your Own: How to Grow Fruit and Vegetables Without Getting Your Hands Too Dirty
By Alex Mitchell (New Holland, 2009)
An essential guide, on growing your own vegetables, fruits, and herbs. Aimed at beginners, it has plenty of practical and seasonal information for planning your edible Eden, delicious recipes, ideas for outdoor entertaining, and fun weekend projects for making your garden look great.

Growing Food in Small Gardens
By Barbara Segall (New Holland, 2012)
Whether you've got a backyard, rooftop, or patio, or are restricted to window boxes or hanging baskets, the joy and satisfaction of organic gardening can be yours. From planning a garden, to deciding what to plant, to the best methods of chemical-free pest and disease control.

How to Grow Food: A Wartime Guide
By Doreen Wallace (Batsford, 2012)
In 1940, Doreen Wallace—novelist, social campaigner, and farmer—wrote *How to Grow Food* as part of Batsford's iconic *Home Front Handbook* series. With its chatty style and beautiful Brian Cook cover, the book became a wartime classic. Gardeners continue to rely on its wisdom today.

The Low Maintenance Vegetable Garden
By Clare Matthews (New Holland, 2010)
Through the simple shortcuts and unconventional low-maintenance strategies presented in this guide, would-be gardeners can learn the tricks needed to grow their own produce without putting in a lot of work. Now even beginners can easily grow fresh fruit and vegetables in their own backyards.

The No-Dig Garden Specialist:
The Essential Guide to Growing Vegetables,
Salads and Soft Fruit in Raised No-Dig Beds
By A. & G. Bridgewater (New Holland, 2011)
For those without the time or stamina to spend hours maintaining a garden, well-known experts Alan and Gill Bridgewater offer an easy-care method with minimal digging and weeding. They show how to make raised beds, build up soil with mushroom compost, cover weeds with mulch, and protect plants with nets and plastic—all using organic methods whenever possible.

The Organic Fruit and Vegetable
Gardener's Year: A Seasonal Guide
to Growing What You Eat
By Graham Clarke
(Guild of Master Craftsman, 2009)
Whether you're planting on a windowsill or in the backyard, *The Organic Fruit and Vegetable Gardener's Year* has the information you need to grow organic produce year-round. Respected horticulture writer Graham Clarke guides gardeners with or without a green thumb through all the basics, from composting and pesticide-free weed control to watering wisely and encouraging pollination.

Organic Gardening: The Whole Story
By Alan & Jackie Gear, foreword by HRH The Prince of Wales (Watkins, 2010)
Organic gardening has blossomed from a humble idea into a global movement. Here, readers will discover the roots of this environmentally conscious approach, from the inspirational story of its two pioneers to the principles behind cultivating produce that is free from pesticides and chemicals. Sprinkled throughout are

encouraging tales of enthusiastic gardeners, from city dwellers to the Prince of Wales himself.

The Organic Vegetable Gardener

By Yvonne Cuthbertson
(Guild of Master Craftsman, 2011)
People today are demanding fresh foods free from toxic chemicals—so this book on growing organic vegetables at home couldn't be timelier. Whether the gardener has a spacious suburban yard or a small city windowsill, all the necessary information and inspiration is here—from choosing the hardiest, most nutritious varieties to harvesting the crop.

COOKBOOKS

Clean Food, Revised Edition
A Seasonal Guide to Eating Close to the Source

Terry Walters (Sterling Epicure, 2012)
Clean Food is a feast for the senses that will nourish mind, body, and soul. Those going gluten-free will find recipe variations throughout the book to meet their needs.

The Garden to Kitchen Expert:
Over 680 Recipes — The Cookery Companion to the World's Best-Selling Gardening Books

By Judith Wills & Dr. D.G. Hessayon
(Expert, 2011)
Now, *The Garden to Kitchen Expert* completes the story, explaining how to prepare all the nutritious produce you have grown for the table. *The Garden to Kitchen Expert* includes: classic recipes for preparing each fruit and vegetable, no-cook methods for serving produce, as well as information on storing, preserving, and pickling what you grow.

Nourish: The Cancer Care Cookbook

By Penny Brohn Cancer Care with Christine Bailey (Duncan Baird; 2013)
Foods, recipes, tools and advice for healing from cancer.

Rose Elliot's New Complete Vegetarian

By Rose Elliot (Sterling, 2010)
As more and more people forego meat, vegetarian cookbooks are the ones "bringing home the bacon." Now, the definitive collection from the "queen of vegetarian cooking" is available again in an exciting new edition.

Superfood Kitchen: Cooking with Nature's Most Amazing Foods

By Julie Morris (Sterling Epicure, 2012)
Beautiful dishes are entirely composed of plant-based, nutrient-dense, and whole foods that energize, nourish, and taste delicious. Each recipe artfully combines natural ingredients that deliver amazing amounts of antioxidants, essential fatty acids (like omega-3), minerals, vitamins, and more.

Superfood Smoothies: 100 Delicious, Energizing & Nutrient-dense Recipes

By Julie Morris (Sterling, 2013)
Nutrient-rich smoothies using the world's most antioxidant-, vitamin-, and mineral-packed foods, and offers innovative culinary

methods for making your smoothies incredibly nutritious and delicious. Whether you're looking for an energy boost, seeking a gentle cleanse, or just trying to get healthy, you'll be inspired to power up the blender!

The 100 Foods You Should Be Eating: How to Source, Prepare and Cook Healthy Ingredients
Glen Matten (New Holland, 2010)
If you listen to all the diet advice out there, the search for healthy foods can become a nightmare. This book is the antidote: a collection of 100 easy-to-prepare recipes—each based on one inexpensive main ingredient—which combine both sound nutrition and mouthwatering taste.

The Top 100 Fitness Foods: 100 Ways to Turbocharge Your Life
By Sarah Owen (Duncan Baird, 2010)
Fit is in! And the first step to getting in shape is taking responsibility for your health. But eating right and following a fitness regime alongside career and family commitments can be a major endurance challenge. *The Top 100 Fitness Foods* is packed with advice on the nutritionally balanced ingredients you need to maximize your energy and achieve your personal best.

Wild About Greens: 125 Delectable Vegan Recipes for Kale, Collards, Arugula, Bok Choy, and other Leafy Veggies Everyone Loves
By Nava Atlas (Sterling, 2012)
Kale, collards, spinach, Asian greens, and many more leafy greens are a breeze to grow and prepare—and these 125 recipes showcase the most commonly used varieties in a wide selection of flavorful dishes.

HISTORY WEB SITES

http://www.foodhistorynews.com/
Run by Food History News, this charming site features lists of public and private food museums, recipes, ingredient (kale, included!) and dish histories, and tons of resources. A must for any foodie!

http://www.foodtimeline.org/
A great place to go and find out when a specific ingredient was first used for food. Kale is included!

http://www.foodreference.com
An excellent source if you're curious about the history of an ingredient, nutrients, or how it is currently used. Yes, kale is included!

http://www.theoldfoodie.com
Type "kale" into the search box and find a number of entertaining articles on the history and historical uses of kale. A fun site!

http://www.oldcook.com/en/index.php
Available in both English and French versions, Old Cook specializes in medieval European gastronomy, but has plenty of information on later food trends. Do a search for "kale" and you'll receive a list of yummy articles.

GARDENING WEB SITES

http://awaytogarden.com/

Beautiful, with a caring, best-friend attitude, A Way To Garden boasts gorgeous photos of everything from veggies, to garden pests (yes, a tomato worm can look pretty) to garden-fresh foods to blog owner Margaret Roach's cats.

http://carletongarden.blogspot.com/

With its breathtaking photos of veggies, gardens, and Skippy the Dog, this site offers up inspiration. Bookmark it so you can easily visit anytime you need to recharge your gardening batteries.

http://chiotsrun.com/

This self-described "chronicle of an organic garden" celebrates food and flower gardening, with chatty posts and beautiful photos.

http://inmykitchengarden.blogspot.com/

Garden lore, advice, photos, and a cornucopia of delicious recipes: This colorful site has it all. Even kale.

http://kgi.org/

The Kitchen Garden International site's tagline is "You can grow your own food. We can help." In fact, the site helps gardeners from Maine to Mumbai, Australia to Austria, young and old. Look up recipes, learn how to preserve your harvest, try saving seeds, and of course, get help in planting the garden of your dreams.

http://mustardplaster.blogspot.com/

Quirky, with an eye for the weird (veggie that is), this humorous site is always good for a laugh, as well as a deeper look at various gardening customs and strange veggies.

http://www.veggiegardener.com/

Another friendly, helpful site that helps even novices grow great veggies. Check out the helpful Troubleshooting and Pest Guides.

http://www.veggiegardeningtips.com/

If you want to grow kale and its brassica cousins, as well as a host of other veggies, this easy-reading site is a must-visit.

http://www.yougrowgirl.com/

Garden writer Gayla Trail's lovely blog. The site celebrates low-cost and no-cost gardening in less-than-ideal spaces. The results are spectacular, as you'll see in the blog's stunning photos.

COOKING WEB SITES

http://www.101cookbooks.com

A terrific site for recipes that use whole food ingredients, including kale.

http://deliciouslyorganic.net

Blogger Carrie Vet's site is filled with yummy, whole food dishes, with a heavy emphasis on veggies (hello, kale!), gluten-free baking, and eating "the paleo way."

http://www.delish.com/

One of the bestblogs for foodies, with menus, food world news, gossip, food shows, and plenty of recipes. Check out the instructions for Kale and Squash Toasts.

http://www.epicurious.com

The behemoth of a site is recipe nirvana for foodies. Upscale, regional, vegan, meat-heavy, ethnic, raw—you name it, there are hundreds of recipes for it, plus travel articles, cooking clinics, restaurant and recipe and product reviews, and more.

http://glutenfreegoddess.blogspot.com/

Lots of wheat-free baking going on at this pretty site. But there are plenty of veggie recipes (many with kale!) as well. Check out the Green Detox Soup, featuring our favorite Brassica.

http://www.healthygreenkitchen.com/

Amaranth, coconut oil, chia, kale, quinoa—we love this blog!

http://www.localharvest.org/

Looking for a local farmer? Farmer's market? CSA? Or simply want to know what's in season in your area? Go to LocalHarvest to find out.

http://www.mydarlinglemonthyme.com

Healthy, gluten-free, veggie-heavy recipes from Perth, Australia. The stunning photos alone make this site one of my favorites.

http://www.sproutedkitchen.com/

Gluten-free, whole foods, pure water, local finds, and recipes that make use of them all. This beautiful site bills itself as "A Tastier Take on Whole Foods."

http://www.mynewroots.blogspot.com/

The tagline for this stunning, veggie-based blog, is "How to Make Health Choices Every Day." Stunning photos with equally stunning recipes (Tandoori Crusted Cauliflower anyone?).

http://www.myrecipes.com

This is a mega-recipe site, with recipes for everything from cakes to kale (320+ of them). It features plenty of smart features, including user reviews, cooking advice, techniques, and the ability to scale a recipe's serving size up or down.

http://ohmyveggies.com/

Enthusiastic and fun (with great recipes) this vegetarian food blog specializes in sophisticated-yet-easy dishes using veggies and fruits.

http://ohsheglows.com/

One woman heals her disorder eating and exercise compulsion, one butternut squash burrito at a time!

http://www.rawfoodrecipes.com

This fun raw cooking site has many interesting-looking (and healthy) kale recipes!

http://www.savvyvegetarian.com

Great, nutrient-dense recipes, many packed with superfoods. Fantastic articles that address all aspect of eating today.

http://www.talkoftomatoes.com

A gardener's cooking blog, Talk of Tomatoes talks candidly of slugs, chickens, kale, and canning.

http://www.theclothesmakethegirl.com/

Melissa Joulwan's funky, irreverent food and

fashion blog is an easy place to lose track of time. A must-see.

http://www.vegkitchen.com/
This is the recipe site of cookbook author Nava Atlas, a woman who knows a lot about cooking greens (kale included) and other veggies. Delicious, easy recipes!

http://www.wholefoodsmarket.com/recipes/
Whole Foods' Web site is loaded with fun recipes—including some with kale!

GENERAL HEALTH WEB SITES

http://www.diet-blog.com
Diet news and research, rolled into one handy blog.

http://www.doctoroz.com/
The good Dr. Oz's Web site.

http://www.eatwellguide.org
Finding local, seasonal food just got easier. Go and plug in our zip code—voila! Farms, markets, restaurants, and more throughout the U.S. and Canada.

http://www.edf.org/
The Environmental Defense Fund's Web site helps individuals avoid environmental pollution in the air, food supply, and everywhere else.

http://www.ewg.org/foodnews/
Environmental Working Group is famous for its regularly updated "dirty dozen" and

"clean fifteen" lists, which help shoppers decide where they can save by purchasing safe mainstream produce, and where it is essential that they go organic.

http://www.fitness.gov
This is the official site for The President's Council on Fitness, Sports & Nutrition.

http://www.foodandwaterwatch.org/blogs/
A look into the politics and players of today's food industries.

http://www.healthfinder.gov
The U.S. government's health site, featuring links, resources, and education.

http://www.mayoclinic.com
The famous Mayo Clinic's health education site.

http://www.mealsmatter.org
The tagline of Meals Matter is "Meal Planning Made Simple." Aimed at busy families and using plenty of familiar (often mainstream) ingredients, this fun site is a great resource for those just easing into a healthier lifestyle.

http://www.medicinenet.com
Easy-to-use source of information on a wide range of conditions, including symptom checkers, and nutritional support.

http://www.naturalnews.com/
NaturalNews is packed with articles, tips, references, videos, podcasts, cartoons, and even music—all in the name of good health.

http://www.patrickholford.com
The UK's answer to Dr. Oz and Dr. Weil, Patrick Holford's sound, practical, holistic nutrition advice helps change lives.

http://www.rodaleinstitute.org
We love Rodale's focus on chemical-free farming, their strong stand against global warming, and the generous nutrition information.

http://www.webmd.com
The authoritative online source of health and slightly holistic medical advice.

http://allfoodsnatural.com/
This pretty site has recipes, natural foods resources and recipes, as well as cooking club to help you upgrade your whole food cooking quotient.

http://www.naturalnews.com/
NaturalNews is packed with articles, tips, references, videos, podcasts, cartoons, and even music—all in the name of good health.

http://www.fruitsandveggiesmatter.gov/
Run by the Centers for Disease Control, this fun, interactive site, makes it easy to get the vegetables and fruits your body needs.

http://greenforlife.com/
Raw food, greens, vegetable smoothies, and more.

http://greensmoothiesblog.com/
Green smoothies are one of the easiest ways to get your veggies. This site is dedicated to the nutrient-dense drink.

http://www.HighImpactHealth.com
Author Stephanie Pedersen's nutrition practice site, with recipes, health advice, and more.

http://www.montereybayaquarium.org/cr/seafoodwatch.aspx
Monterey Bay Aquarium's famous "Seafood Watch" helps consumers choose safe, low-metal seafood that is not endangered. Good for your body, good for the planet.

http://www.nutritionalresearch.org/
Packed full with links to nutrition research studies, as well as other resources. A must-visit site!

www.StephaniePedersen.com
Site of Stephanie Pedersen, author of *Kale: The Complete Guide to the World's Most Powerful Superfood.*

www.superfoodsrx.com
This commercial site has a plethora of information on favorite high-impact foods, as well as nutrients, a collection of research, and an up-to-the-minute blog.

http://userealbutter.com/
This gorgeous, tasty site espouses eating real foods, including superfoods such as kale, chia, and quinoa. Fantastic recipes.

http://www.whfoods.com
Billing itself as "the world's healthiest foods," WHFoods.com is an awesome collection of whole, super and functional foods, with

plenty of research studies, nutrient profiles, allergy info, habitat, history, and cultural background for each food. Highly recommended.

http://witchenkitchen.com/
Herbs—eating them, healing with them, growing them, picking them!

PUBLICATIONS

www.cleaneatingmag.com
Clean Eating is a newcomer to the world of magazines. It is aimed at taking you beyond the food you eat to explore the multitude of health and nutritional benefits of living a clean lifestyle.

http://www.cookinglight.com
A favorite of calorie counters and long-term dieters, *Cooking Light* makes your favorite foods less caloric.

http://www.eatingwell.com
One of our favorite magazines, *Eating Well* talks health from the plate up. Filled with whole foods recipes, health articles, research, and personal essays.

http://www.fitnessmagazine.com
Fitness magazine has all kinds of exercise and get-fit advice, with a healthy dose of diet and nutrition information.

http://www.health.com
General health magazine with a fitness and diet focus.

http://www.livingwithout.com
Living Without is the go-to resource for anyone living with food allergies, sensitivities, or intolerances. Filled with cutting-edge research, as well as in-depth looks at specific food issues, it also features loads of wheat-free, dairy-free and soy-free recipes, many of them containing chia.

http://www.mensfitness.com
With a strong emphasis on sculpting the body through weight lifting and exercise, *Men's Fitness* also has diet and nutrition advice.

http://www.menshealth.com
Published by Rodale Press, *Men's Health* is a mainstream fitness-oriented magazine with plenty of nutrition and weight loss advice.

http://www.naturalhealthmag.com
What began as a "hardcore" macrobiotic and spirituality publication, has recently gone mainstream with advice on everything from mindset to healthy eating to green living.

http://www.prevention.com
Another Rodale Press publication, *Prevention* is the time-honored source of research-based diet, exercise, lifestyle and nutrition information.

http://www.vegetariantimes.com
Vegetarian Times tagline is "Great Food, Good Health, Smart Living," which is what this fun, informative magazine is all about.

www.vegnews.com
This magazine is aimed at hardcore vegans—but its health articles and recipes are great for everyone.

http://www.womenshealthmag.com
Published by Rodale Press, *Women's Health* is a mainstream fitness-oriented magazine with plenty of nutrition and weight loss advice.

http://www.wholeliving.com
Created by the publishers of *Martha Stewart Living*, this fun magazine has a green bent, which colors everything from its recipes to its fashion sections.

ORGANIZATIONS
http://www.eatright.org/
American Dietetic Association is not the most progressive food education organization around, but it provides solid information on basic nutrition.

http://www.eco-farm.org/
Nurturing healthy farms, food systems, and communities.

http://www.farmtoschool.org
Farm to School connects schools (K–12) and local farms with the objectives of serving healthy meals in school cafeterias, improving student nutrition, providing agriculture, health and nutrition education opportunities, and supporting local and regional farmers.

http://www.nutrition.org/
The American Society for Nutrition stands for excellence in nutrition research and science.

www.nourishingtheplanet.org
WorldWatch Institute's Nourish The Planet program is a nonprofit focused on highlighting environmentally sustainable ways of alleviating hunger and poverty.

http://www.organicconsumers.org/
The organic Consumers Association helps maintain organic food standards.

http://www.panna.org/
Pesticide Action Network provides information about harmful pesticides and works to replace pesticide use with ecologically sound and socially just alternatives.

http://www.slowfood.com/
Slow Food works to preserve traditional, cultural foods, recipes and ways of eating.

http://www.sustainabletable.org
Sustainable Table celebrates local sustainable food and growing methods.

http://truefoodnow.org/
The True Food Network's Center for Food Safety works to protect human health and the environment by curbing the proliferation of harmful food production technologies and by promoting organic and other forms of sustainable agriculture.

INDEX

Note: Page numbers *in italics* indicate recipes.

Anti-inflammatory benefits
  fruits, 35, 36, 45, 101, 108
  herbs, 44, 63, 113
  kale/kale ingredients, 6, 16, 24, 26, 27, 42, 157, 158, 159
  olives and olive oil, 83, 127
  omega-3s, omega-6s and, 26, 27
  onions, 52
Antioxidants
  about, 11, 48
  examples of, 20, 21, 23, 30, 35, 41, 55, 63, 94, 97, 123, 127, 131, 133. *See also* Flavonoids
  kale juice and, 42
Appetizers and snacks, 105–119
  dips, 118–119
    Garlicky Kale and Spinach Dip, *119*
    Green Surprise Dip, *119*
    Lemon-Ricotta Kale Dip, *118*
  kale and fruit snacks, 107–110
    Kale Cacao Energy Truffles, *107–108*
    Kale Cheese Dates, *108*
    Kale Granola Bars, *108–110*
  kale chips and crackers, 105–107
    about: making chips, 162–163
    Baked Kale Chips, *106*
    Kale Crackers, *105*
    Salt and Vinegar Kale Chips, *107*
  savories, 111–117
    Baked Feta with Kale Pesto on Baguette, *113*
    Chicken and Kale Hand Pies, *112–113*
    Kale and Bean Bruschetta, *114*
    Kale and Gorgonzola Swirls, *111*
    Kale Mini Pizzas, *114*
    Pickled Kale—The Perfect Condiment, *117*
    Spinach and Kale Turnovers, *116*
    Squash-and-Kale Toasts, *116–117*
Apples
  about: making applesauce, 149
  Apple and Kale Spice Muffins, *65*
  Refreshing Kale Cooler, *44*
  Sunshine Juice, *46*
  Warming Autumn Kale Juice, *48*

Arthritis, 159. *See also* Anti-inflammatory benefits
Avocados
  about: characteristics and benefits, 35; latex allergies and, 35
  Green Goddess Pudding, *146–147*
  Mint Dessert Shake, *34–35*

Bananas
  about: benefits and characteristics, 39
  Banana Kale Smoothie, *38*
  Vegan Banana-Kale Muffins, *70*
Barley-Kale Stew, *81–82*
Beans and legumes
  about: cannellini beans, 84; garbanzos/chickpeas, 86, 102–103; lentils, 87; preparation pointers, 89
  Cannellini-Butternut-Kale Stew, *83*
  Chicken with Kale Lentil Pilaf, *122–123*
  Chickpea and Kale Sandwich Spread or Salad, *102*
  Garbanzo Kale Soup, *86*
  Good Karma Sandwich, *99*
  Green Surprise Dip, *119*
  Kale and Bean Bruschetta, *114*
  Kale and Cannellini Soup, *84–85*
  Kaled-Up Split Pea Soup, *89*
  Lentil and Vegetable Stew with Kale, *86–87*
  Pinto-Bean Mole Chili, *90*
Beets, *44*, *48*, 155
Benefits of kale, 5–6, 157–159. *See also* Anti-inflammatory benefits; Nutrients, kale
Berries
  about: strawberries, 36
  Blueberry Kale Pops, *143–144*
  Kale Berry Blast, *36–37*
  Red Kale Juice, *44*
  Super Awesome Health Muffins, *69*
  Superfood Protein Smoothie, *40–41*
Beta-carotene, 6. *See also* Vitamin A
Black pepper, 78
Bloat, losing, *43*
Brassica family, 5, 11, 13, 92–93, 119
Brassica napus or oleracea, 11, 12
Breads. *See* Breakfast; Sandwiches

Breakfast, 51–79. *See also* Eggs
  about: kale with, 51
  cereal, 71–72
    about: nutritional benefits of oats, 72
    Irish Oats, *71*
  Chorizo Kale Hash Browns, *76*
  hotcakes, 73–75
    about: pancakes, 73; waffles, 74, 75
    Dinner-Style Kale Pancakes, *73*
    Kale Waffles, *74*
    Savory Waffles, *74–75*
  muffins, 65–71
    about: baking without gluten, 67; fast and easy, 66;
      sugar in, 71; trivia, 70; whole wheat pastry flour for, 71;
      vegan "buttermilk," 65
    Apple and Kale Spice Muffins, *65*
    Morning Glory Kale Muffins, *66*
    Savory Carrot and Kale Muffins (grain-free/gluten-free), *67*
    Summer Squash-Kale Muffins, *68–69*
    Super Awesome Health Muffins, *69*
    Vegan Banana-Kale Muffins, *70*
  potatoes, 76–79
    about: hash browns, 76; preparation options, 77
    Kale, Potato, and Onion Frittata, *56–57*
    Oven Hash Kale Cakes, *77*
    Potato and Kale Galette, *78–79*
  sandwiches, 62–64
    about: bread for, 64; tartines, 65
    Bacon, Kale, and Sweet Potato Breakfast Burritos, *62*
    Everything Kale Breakfast Sandwich, *63*
    Kale Tartine, *64*
Brussels sprouts, *92–93*, 164
Bulgur, *96*
Burritos, breakfast, 62
"Buttermilk," vegan, 65
Buying kale, 10

Calcium, 28, 97, 100, 157, 159
Carotenoids, 22–23, 35, 41, 53, 75, 101, 158
Carrots
  Savory Carrot and Kale Muffins (grain-free/gluten-free), *67*
  Warming Autumn Kale Juice, *48*
Casserole, kale, *136–137*
Celery
  about: benefits of, 44
  Kale Waldorf Salad, *98*
  Lose the Bloat Kale Drink, *43*
  Roasted Red Pepper-Kale Strata, *60*

Cheese
  Baked Feta with Kale Pesto on Baguette, *113*
  Kale and Gorgonzola Swirls, *111*
  Kale Cheese Dates, *108*
  Kale Mini Pizzas, *114*
  Lemon-Ricotta Kale Dip, *118*
  Spicy Kale-Cheese Sandwich, *99*
Chia, *40–41*
Chicken
  about: arsenic in, 122
  Chicken and Kale Hand Pies, *112–113*
  Chicken Kale Braise, *121–122*
  Chicken with Kale Lentil Pilaf, *122–123*
  Spicy Chicken Kale Stir-Fry, *131*
Chips and crackers. *See* Appetizers and snacks; Chocolate;
  Desserts and other sweets
Chocolate
  about: cacao nibs, 148; cacao vs. cocoa, 34: Devil's Food, 155
  Choco-Kale Health Shake, *34*
  Chocolate Surprise Granola Clusters, *144–145*
  Cocoa-Dusted Kale Chips, *145*
  Deep Chocolate-Cloaked Kale Chips, *146*
  Kale Cacao Energy Truffles, *107–108*
  Kaled-Up Boxed Mix Brownies, *147*
  Kaled-Up Chocolate Brownies (from scratch), *149–150*
  Nutty Choco-Kale Shake, *36*
  Vegan Cocoa-Kale Cupcakes, *152*
  Wicked Kale Cupcakes, *155*
Cholesterol
  fiber and, 25, 159
  foods aiding levels, 41, 47, 58, 63, 68, 83, 85, 98, 108, 127
    minerals and, 28, 30
Chorizo. *See* Pork
Cilantro, about, 63
Cinnamon, benefits, 68
Citrus
  about: easy lemon zest, 69; lemon juice, 117
  Kale Lime Slushy, *38*
  Lemon-Ricotta Kale Dip, *118*
  Sunshine Juice, *46*
Coconut products, about, 150–151
Cooking FAQs, 162–164
Copper, 28, 29, 55, 72, 78, 87, 98, 108, 133, 157, 159
Copper pots, 29
Creamed Kale, *132*
Creamy Kale Smoothie, 37
Cruciferous family, 12

Cucumbers
  Refreshing Kale Cooler, *44*
  Stay-Well Kale Juice, *45*
  Stephanie's Build-Your-Own Kale Smoothie Blueprint, *40*
Cumin, 123

Dandelion leaves, *43*
Dates
  about, 108, 109
  Kale Cacao Energy Truffles, *107–108*
  Kale Cheese Dates, *108*
Desserts and other sweets, 143–155. *See also* Chocolate
  about: coconut products and, 150–151; decorating cupcakes,
    153; making applesauce, 149; nutty topper, 147
  Blueberry Kale Pops, *143–144*
  Dessert Chips (Kale-Style), *146*
  Green Goddess Pudding, *146–147*
  Vegan Juicer-Pulp Muffin, *153–154*
Detoxifying, 6, 24, 25, 40, 48, 63, 117, 157
Diabetes, 52, 64, 159. *See also* Glycemic index chart
Dinner, 121–141
  about: kale with, 121
  entrees, 121–131. *See also* Pasta
    Chicken Kale Braise, *121–122*
    Chicken with Kale Lentil Pilaf, *122–123*
    Kale Mushroom Polenta, *124–125*
    Kale-Pork Gratin, *126*
    Pork Chops with Kale Chip Gremolata, *129–130*
    Spicy Chicken Kale Stir-Fry, *131*
  side dishes, 132–141
    Creamed Kale, *132*
    Fried Pork Rice with Kale, *134*
    Green Polenta, *133*
    Green Potato Puree, *135*
    Hearty Winter Salad, *136*
    Kale Casserole, *136–137*
    Kale Meat Pies, *138*
    Kale Rice, *138–139*
    Potato Kale Cakes, *140*
    Potliker Kale, *141*
Dips, 118–119
Diverticulitis, 166
Dreams, vitamin B6 and, 19
Drinks
  about: kale in, 33
  juices, 42–49
    about: celery in, 44; diluting or not, 42; drinking immediately,
      48; garlic in, 47; ginger in, 44; juicers for, 45; kale

straight up, 42; parsley in, 43; pineapple in, 45; pulp
      uses, 154; sugar/glycemic index and, 46; tomatoes in, 47
    Lose the Bloat Kale Drink, *43*
    Red Kale Juice, *44*
    Refreshing Kale Cooler, *44*
    Stay-Well Kale Juice, *45*
    Sunshine Juice, *46*
    V8-Style Juice, *47*
    Vegan Juicer-Pulp Muffin, *153–154*
    Warming Autumn Kale Juice, *48*
  shakes, 34–36
    Choco-Kale Health Shake, *34*
    Mint Dessert Shake, *34–35*
    Nutty Choco-Kale Shake, *36*
  smoothies, 36–42
    about: kale for, 164; making, 38; on the road, 42
    Banana Kale Smoothie, *38*
    Creamy Kale Smoothie, *37*
    Kale Berry Blast, *36–37*
    Kale Lime Slushy, *38*
    Stephanie's Build-Your-Own Kale Smoothie Blueprint, *40*
    Superfood Protein Smoothie, *40–41*
    Tropical Smoothie, *41*

Eggs
  about: 56; nutritional benefits, 57, 59; making omelets, 59;
    quiches, 59; safety and handling, 61; vegan replacement, 66
  Breakfast Casserole, *51–52*
  Everything Kale Breakfast Sandwich, *63*
  Kale-Bacon Quiche Cups, *53*
  Kale-Mushroom-Poblano Frittata, *54–55*
  Kale, Potato, and Onion Frittata, *56–57*
  Kale Tartine, *64*
  Poached Eggs with Kale-Chorizo Hash, *57*
  Quiche with Kale, *58–59*
  Roasted Red Pepper-Kale Strata, *60*
  Scrambled Kale Eggs, *60–61*
Energy, kale providing, 5
Eye health, 23

Farro, *96*
Fiber
  benefits and characteristics, 24–25
  diverticulitis and, 166
  for indigestion, 25
  kale and, 6, 24–25
  soluble vs. insoluble, 25, 158–159

Flavonoids, 24, 43, 52, 53, 58, 101, 108, 148, 157
Folate or folic acid. See Vitamin B9 (folate or folic acid)
Frequently asked questions, 157–167
    cooking with kale, 162–164
    growing kale, 159–162
    history of kale, 164–165
    nutrients and benefits, 157–159
    safety considerations, 166–167
Fruit. See Appetizers and snacks; specific fruit

Gallbladder and gallstones, 6, 19, 101
Garlic, about, 119
Ginger, about, 44, 110
Glucosinolates, 24, 157
Gluten, baking without, 67
Glycemic index chart, 46
Granola, 108–110, 144–145
Gratin, 126
Growing kale, 159–162, 169–173

Heart health, 6, 16, 27, 55, 75, 158
Heart rate, 28, 30, 31
Hotcakes. See Breakfast

Immune system function
    kale/kale nutrients and, 6, 21, 22, 26, 42
    other foods aiding, 43, 44, 47, 52, 53, 83, 108, 144
    vitamins aiding, 36, 41, 58, 85
Iron, 78
    about, 28–29
    aids in metabolizing, 17, 28
    deficiency, 29
    forms of, 29
    functions of, 28
    sources of, 72, 78, 84, 87, 97, 103, 108, 123, 129, 133

Joint health, 6
Juices. See Drinks

Kale
    author's experience, 4–7
    benefits, 5–6, 157–159. See also Anti-inflammatory benefits;
        Nutrients, kale; specific vitamins and minerals
    choosing/buying, 10, 165
    cooking time, 111
    cooking with, FAQs, 162–164
    FAQs, 157–167
    growing, 159–162, 169–173
    history of, 9, 10, 164–165

leaf quality, 10
other names for, 11
popularity of, 6–7
pre-prepping, 11
recipes. See Appetizers and snacks; Desserts and other sweets;
    Drinks; specific main ingredients (non-kale); specific meals
safety considerations, 166–167
Scotland and, 96, 100, 111, 135, 165
storing, 10–11, 12, 165–166
tastes/flavors of, 5, 9
types and varieties, 4–5, 9–10, 11, 12, 161
washing, 10–11, 12
wilt, avoiding/reviving, 10, 165–166
Kale Queens, 164–165

Leeks, 58–59
Lemon or lime. See Citrus
Lunch, kale with, 81. See also Salads; Sandwiches; Soups,
    stews, and chilis
Lutein, 23, 101
Lycopene, 75

Magnesium, 30, 72, 85, 97, 98, 108
Manganese, 30, 36, 40, 52, 78, 85, 87, 97, 98, 108, 159
Mangos, 41
Maple syrup
    about: marvels of, 40
    Stephanie's Build-Your-Own Kale Smoothie Blueprint, 40
    Superfood Protein Smoothie, 40–41
Metals, detoxing. See Detoxifying
Mint, 34–35, 40, 45
Muffins, other. See Breakfast
Muffins, vegan juicer-pulp, 153–154
Mushrooms
    about, 55, 124
    Kale-Mushroom-Poblano Frittata, 54–55
    Kale Mushroom Polenta, 124–125

Niacin. See Vitamin B3 (niacin)
Nutrients, kale, 15–31. See also specific vitamins and minerals
    about: overview of, 5
    benefits summary, 5–6
    FAQs, 157–159
    optimizing, 11
Nuts and seeds
    about: cashew trivia, 37; chestnut health benefits, 85; dessert
        topper, 147; making nut butter, 36; peanut power, 94;
        pine nuts, 97; sesame oil, 131; sesame seeds, 98; tahini, 136;
        walnut lore, 144

Creamy Kale Smoothie, *37*
Kale Cacao Energy Truffles, *107–108*
Nuts-and-Seeds Kale Salad, *97*
Nutty Choco-Kale Shake, *36*
Nutty Kale Slaw, *93–94*
Superfood Protein Smoothie, *40–41*

Oats
  about: nutritional benefits, 72
  Chocolate Surprise Granola Clusters, *144–145*
  Irish Oats, *71*
  Kale Granola Bars, *108–110*
Olives and olive oil, 83, 127, 128
Omega-3 essential fatty acids
  benefits of, 26, 159
  changing diets and, 27
  from kale, 5–6, 26, 158, 159
  other sources of, 26, 59
Omega-6 essential fatty acids, 27, 59, 158
Onions, 52, *56–57*
Oxalates, 19, 166

Pancakes, *73*
Parsley
  about: nutritional benefits, 43, 129
  Lose the Bloat Kale Drink, *43*
  Stephanie's Build-Your-Own Kale Smoothie Blueprint, *40*
Pasta
  Fast Fettuccine with Kale and Sausage, *127*
  Nona's Pasta, *125*
  One-Pot Green Penne, *128–129*
Pears, *48*, 101, *101*
Pepper, black, 78
Peppers
  about: nutritional benefits, 53
  Kale-Bacon Quiche Cups, *53*
  Kale-Mushroom-Poblano Frittata, *54–55*
  Nutty Kale Slaw, *93–94*
  Roasted Red Pepper-Kale Strata, *60*
Pesto, kale, *113*
Phosphorous, 31, 47, 95, 103, 157
Pickled Kale—The Perfect Condiment, *117*
Pies, savory, *112–113*, 138
Pineapple, *45*
Pizza, *114*, 115
Polenta, green, *133*
Pork
  about: chorizo/sausage, 88; made healthy, 126

Bacon, Kale, and Sweet Potato Breakfast Burritos, *62*
Caramelized Shallot-Kale-Prosciutto Sandwich, *100*
Chorizo Kale Hash Browns, *76*
Fast Fettuccine with Kale and Sausage, *127*
Fried Pork Rice with Kale, *134*
Kale-Bacon Quiche Cups, *53*
Kale Meat Pies, *138*
Kale-Pork Gratin, *126*
Poached Eggs with Kale-Chorizo Hash, *57*
Pork Chops with Kale Chip Gremolata, *129–130*
Pork Pumpkin Stew, *90–91*
Potato Soup with Kale and Chorizo, *87–88*
Potassium, 39, 47, 55, 85, 87, 95, 97, 108, 133, 157
Potatoes
  about: consumption statistics, 135; hash browns, 76; history in America, 141; preparation options, 77
  Chorizo Kale Hash Browns, *76*
  Green Potato Puree, *135*
  Hearty Winter Salad, *136*
  Kale, Potato, and Onion Frittata, *56–57*
  Oven Hash Kale Cakes, *77*
  Potato and Kale Galette, *78–79*
  Potato Kale Cakes, *140*
  Potato Soup with Kale and Chorizo, *87–88*
Pre-prepping kale, 11
Protein
  about, 26–27
  animal sources, 88, 127
  chia for, 41
  complete vs. incomplete, 27
  in desserts, 146
  kale for, 27
  other sources, 36, 37, 72, 84, 94, 95, 96
  recipes featuring, *40–41*, *60–61*, *86–87*, *96*, *97*, *107–108*
Pumpkin, in Pork Pumpkin Stew, *90–91*
Pumpkin seeds, 91

Quinoa
  Chicken with Kale Lentil Pilaf, *122–123*
  Kale Quinoa Salad, *96*
  Nuts-and-Seeds Kale Salad, *97*

Recipes. See Appetizers and snacks; Desserts and other sweets; Drinks; *specific main ingredients (non-kale)*; *specific meals*
Resources, 174–183
Riboflavin. See Vitamin B2 (riboflavin)
Rice
  about, 139

Chicken with Kale Lentil Pilaf, *122–123*
Kale Rice, *138–139*
Rosemary, 113

Safety, kale and, 166–167
Salads, 92–98
    Basic Kale Salad, *92*
    Brassica Salad, *92–93*
    Butternut Squash and Kale Salad, *94–95*
    Chickpea and Kale Sandwich Spread or Salad, *102*
    Hearty Winter Salad, *136*
    Kale Quinoa Salad, *96*
    Kale Waldorf Salad, *98*
    Nuts-and-Seeds Kale Salad, *97*
    Nutty Kale Slaw, *93–94*
Sandwiches, 99–103. *See also* Breakfast
    Caramelized Shallot-Kale-Prosciutto Sandwich, *100*
    Chickpea and Kale Sandwich Spread or Salad, *102*
    Good Karma Sandwich, *99*
    Spicy Kale-Cheese Sandwich, *99*
    Turkey Orchard Sandwich, *101*
Sausage. *See* Pork
Seeds. *See* Nuts and seeds
Sesame oil, 131
Shakes. *See* Drinks
Shallots, *100*, 133
Side dishes. *See* Dinner
Skin health
    kale/kale nutrients and, 5, 17, 18, 20, 26, 28, 164
    olive oil and, 128
    omega-3s, omega-6s and, 26, 158
Sleep, kale and, 19, 31
Smoothies. *See* Drinks
Snacks. *See* Appetizers and snacks
Soups, stews, and chilis, 81–91
    about: barley nutrition, 82
    Barley-Kale Stew, *81–82*
    Cannellini-Butternut-Kale Stew, *83*
    Garbanzo Kale Soup, *86*
    Kale and Cannellini Soup, *84–85*
    Kaled-Up Split Pea Soup, *89*
    Lentil and Vegetable Stew with Kale, *86–87*
    Pinto-Bean Mole Chili, *90*
    Pork Pumpkin Stew, *90–91*
    Potato Soup with Kale and Chorizo, 87–88
Soy sauce, sodium and, 134
Spinach, *116*, *119*

Squash
    about: butternut, 95
    Butternut Squash and Kale Salad, *94–95*
    Cannellini-Butternut-Kale Stew, *83*
    Pinto-Bean Mole Chili, *90*
    Squash-and-Kale Toasts, *116–117*
    Summer Squash-Kale Muffins, *68–69*
Storing kale, 10–11, 12, 165–166
Stuttering, 16
Sweet potatoes, *48*, *62*

Thiamin. *See* Vitamin B1 (thiamin)
Thyme, 113
Tomatoes, 47
Toxins, removing. *See* Detoxifying
Tryptophan, 31, 87, 157
Turkey, *101*, 127

Vegan foods
    about: buttermilk substitution, 65; egg replacement, 66
    Garlicky Kale and Spinach Dip, *119*
    Kale and Bean Bruschetta, *114*
    Vegan Banana-Kale Muffins, *70*
    Vegan Cocoa-Kale Cupcakes, *152*
    Vegan Juicer-Pulp Muffin, *153–154*
Vinegar, 100, *107*
Vitamin A, 6, 10, 15–16, 41, 43, 53, 58, 95, 129
Vitamin B1 (thiamin), 16, 72, 85, 87, 98
Vitamin B2 (riboflavin), 17, 55, 85
Vitamin B3 (niacin), 17–18, 55, 85
Vitamin B6, 18–19, 41
Vitamin B9 (folate or folic acid), 19–20, 85, 87, 129
Vitamin C, 10, 20–21, 36, 41, 43, 45, 52, 58, 85, 101, 129, 159, 165
Vitamin E, 21, 58, 97, 144
Vitamin K, 21–22, 35, 43, 58, 78, 101, 129, 157

Waffles, *74–75*
Washing kale, 10–11, 12
Weight loss, 158
Wilt, avoiding/reviving, 10, 165–166

Yogurt
    about: coconut, 151
    Green Surprise Dip, *119*
    Super Awesome Health Muffins, *69*

Zeaxanthin, 23, 101
Zucchini. *See* Squash

ABOUT THE AUTHOR

Stephanie Pedersen, MS, CHHC, AADP, is a holistic nutritionist. A speaker and author of more than 20 books, Stephanie has a reputation for giving her clients the edge they need to get whatever they want from life. She does this by helping individuals to lose weight, manage food allergies, and detoxify naturally, using food and lifestyle changes.

As Stephanie says, "I want health for everyone! I have seen firsthand with myself and my own clients that when one works to get clean and fit and address your health challenges, life gets bigger. Suddenly, life becomes outrageously fun and easy. You move healthfully through life with ease."

According to Stephanie, getting healthy doesn't have to be complicated, or time-consuming. "As a mother, a writer, a nutritionist, a PTA mom, and someone who loves to have time alone to wander local farmer's markets, I know that complicated, overly-fussy diets, or an unnatural obsession with calorie-counting, are not the answers to getting and staying healthy." Instead, Stephanie espouses a life of love, laughter, daily exercise, and your favorite whole foods. (Including plenty of kale!) "We're lucky that we live in a time when more and more gorgeous whole food ingredients, organic produce, and humanely farmed meat is available. Let's celebrate our good fortunate by exploring our many food and fitness options and experimenting with abandon!"

Pedersen currently lives in New York City with her husband and three sons. Visit her at **www.StephaniePedersen.com**

Also by Stephanie Pedersen:

KISS Guide to Beauty: Keep It Simple Series

Ginseng: Energy Enhancer

Garlic: Safe and Effective Self-Care for Arthritis, High Blood Pressure, and Flu

Bra: A Thousand Years of Style, Support and Seduction

ACKNOWLEDGMENTS

I couldn't have finished *Kale: The Complete Guide To The World's Most Powerful Superfood* without the support of my husband, Richard Joseph Demler, and our sons Leif Christian Pedersen, Anders Gyldenvalde Pedersen and Axel SuneLund Pedersen. Thank you to the DreamKeepers: Katy Terpack Tafoya, Michele Grace Lessirard, Marlowe Aster, Vicky White, Ann Brosnan, Sherri McLendon. Though we're scattered across the globe, you are always here. I think of you as sisters. Thanks, too, to the NYC wellness community, which is a surprisingly tight-knit, happy group of healers, who have reminded me to have fun as I lived (ate, cooked, and wrote) kale for several months!

Thanks to my amazing clients for the constant inspiration they bring. Every day I am amazed at your drive, your courage, and your will. Getting healthy can be scary, and yet you see the joy in being healthy, dive in, and create vibrant good health for yourself. Yay, you! I am in awe of each of you. I happen to have been working with a group of detoxers (hello, 21-Day Power Life detoxers!!!) during the last stretch of the *Kale* manuscript and it couldn't have been better timing: Raw kale salad, kale smoothies, kale chips, kale green juice—all were springboards for fabulous detox conversations! I've never had so much fun during a detox program or writing a book!

I can't say enough flattering things about my editor, Kate Zimmermann, and my other Sterling Publishing friends, Jennifer Williams and Barbara Berger. My book producer, Laurie Dolphin and her designer Allison Meierding ensured that the finished product was as polished and professional as possible. Your calm, can-do demeanors and overall smarty-pants ways, make this crazy business of publishing look glamorous. Bill Milne created the gorgeous, mouth-watering food photos in *Kale*. Thank you!

Thanks, too, to every kale grower—whether commercial farmer or backyard gardener—who has ever lived. Without you, there would be no kale chips. No kale smoothies. No *grønkålssuppe*. The world would be a less green, less healthy place. Lastly, I must thank you, dear reader and kale lover, for your interest. Thank you!

PHOTOGRAPHY CREDITS